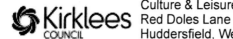
England. Trained as a ___ studied further in medical research at a leading British children's hospital specialising in neurological disorders. When Renée was twenty-one she was involved in a serious car accident that kept her in an English hospital for nearly two years. Wheelchair-bound with a lively toddler to raise, she beat the odds and walked again.

Renée returned to Sydney in 1967, and taught children with disabilities. Subsequently she was lecturer in French at the NSW State Conservatorium of Music and French language coach for the Australian Opera. In 1980 she joined SBSTV, where she worked as administrator, editor and translator for twelve years.

Renée spent nine years living in France and England and wrote for newspapers and magazines. She now lives in Sydney. Her memoir *Belonging* was published in 2003.

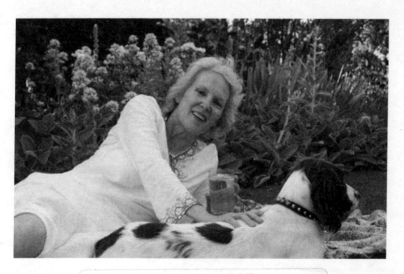

Pain Management

ENHANCING YOUR LIFE TO THE FULLEST

Renée Goossens

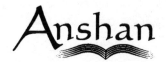

For my son Philip Alexander

First published in the UK by
Anshan Ltd
in 2009

11a Little Mount Sion
Tunbridge Wells
Kent. TN1 1YS

Tel: +44 (0) 1892 557767
Fax: +44 (0) 1892 530358
E-mail: info@anshan.co.uk
www.anshan.co.uk

ISBN 978 1848290 099

British Library Cataloguing in Publication Data
A catalogue record for this book is available from the British Library

Printed by Athenaeum Press, UK

10 9 8 7 6 5 4 3 2 1

This book is dedicated to the memory of
Harry Pickering
5 July 1994–17 November 2000

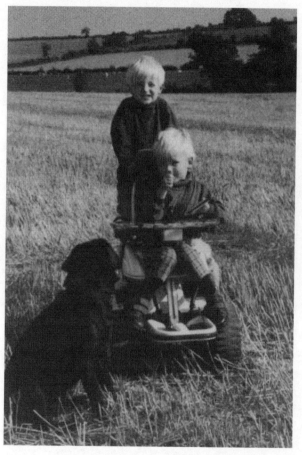

Harry Pickering & brother Cameron
with dog Pingu

Contents

Foreword

This book is extraordinary in that it is written by a patient for patients. In compiling research, the author undertook over one hundred interviews with families in Australia, France and England, following up some of these patients and their families for up to five years. She also sought the advice of numerous medical and other health professionals from a wide range of disciplines. To this she brings her personal perspective, as one who has successfully fulfilled roles as mother, teacher, translator, writer and a great friend to many in the face of increasing physical disability and severe pain.

Renée Goossens knows at first hand that there is more to the expdrience of chronic pain than the pain itself. Her book deals with associated problems such as fatigue, difficulty in concentrating, loss of confidence, anxiety and depression. It stresses the suffering, both physical and emotional, of the whole family when one of its members is unwell and unable to participate in usual activities. It contains practical, commonsense advice. It is a book that can be read in large segments or dipped into occasionally.

It is unusual for a subject of such breadth and complexity to be presented from a non-medical point of view, and it is difficult to achieve a balance of readability and rigour. No one is better equipped to do so than Renée Goossens, and she has successfully risen to the challenge in this book.

Richard Hallinan, FAChAM (RACP)

Prologue

Renée's Story, Part I

Late winter, 1962, Berkshire, England. It was a freak accident. According to the police report, a soft-top Morris Minor 1000 had jumped a country hedgerow, thrown all the passengers out into a field, rolled three times, leaving deep indentations in the grass, then had come to a stop on top of the body of a young woman.

The wreckage was out of sight. Two hours later a couple in a passing car heard the sound of a baby crying. The woman insisted they search for the baby. What they found about a hundred metres away was a field strewn with three bodies — a woman in her late fifties, a young man in his early twenties, both of whom were unconscious, and a baby in a carrycot crying and hungry but miraculously unhurt — and an overturned car with an arm protruding from beneath it. The woman ran to a nearby house to call an ambulance. The man remained at the scene of the accident clutching the outstretched hand.

The two adults who had been flung into the field regained

consciousness as the first ambulance arrived. The man crouching beside the car kept holding the hand poking out from beneath the wreck. An army colonel, from his knowledge of first aid he knew that the young woman required a doctor and probably an immediate transfusion of intravenous fluids. He stretched beneath the car and measured the weakening pulse of the bloodless arm. The woman was unconscious and barely breathing, but she kept a tight grip on the colonel's hand. He hoped that if he could keep hold of her till the moment she was taken into the operating theatre somehow this link might keep her alive.

The ambulance driver radioed for back-up medical staff and arranged for a crane driver to move the car's weight from the young woman. It was a skilful task: the slightest incorrect move-ment could cause her death. The team arrived almost an hour later.

The three passengers in the first ambulance were checked out as fit at the hospital. The woman's crushed ribs were strapped, as was the usual practice then. The young man was concussed, stunned and fearful about his wife — picturing her in the field beneath the car. The seven-month-old baby had settled well in the arms of a nurse, who gave him a warmed bottle of milk. He was sleeping soundly by the time the second ambulance arrived with the young woman, identified as his mother.

The headline in the *Oxford Times* of 20 February 1962 read: 'Mother Killed Baby Lives in Freak Accident'.

The newspaper was wrong. I was that young woman.

My pelvis was fractured in nine places and the fractured bones had caused internal organ damage. My liver had burst and, as the surgeon noted, 'it was as if a bomb had exploded' within my body. My bowel, spleen, bladder and womb were also damaged: repairs were sutured where possible, the liver reconstructed as best could be, the spleen removed, and blood transfusions of twelve litres administered over the following three days. I was unconscious for three and a half weeks. But at one point, I distinctly heard a doctor say, 'This one won't last twenty-four hours.' A voice within me wanted to scream in language I seldom use, 'I'll bloody fight and live, you'll see.' I had a young baby to care for and a husband who loved me.

When I regained consciousness, I spoke only in French (which I knew well, but it was not my first language). The doctors thought I was rambling nonsense until a physiotherapist who came in to assist my breathing said, 'That's not nonsense, it's French. She's asking where she is.'

True, I did believe I was on another planet. Just before the crash, we had been listening to the radio broadcast about John Glenn going into space.

It took eighteen months to get out of the Radcliffe Infirmary. My first operation had taken over nine hours. I had been lucky. I was alive. But all agreed that I would never walk again. I was twenty-one, and this was very hard to cope with. Terrified that my baby might be taken from me forever — he was with my husband's parents during my hospital stay — I was determined to prove everyone wrong. When I left hospital I was still in a wheelchair, yet more certain than ever to disprove what I regarded as their 'curse'.

At times like this it seems we either fight harder — if there is something we can fight for — or we give in. One of the reasons

I am writing this book is to demonstrate there is always something worth fighting for.

Probably most of us have an opportunity in our lifetime to learn something very important and, if we don't take that lesson, we keep receiving it again, until finally we get the point. I learned to fight to live, to recover, to keep going — come what may. The period in hospital was one in which I became virtually institutionalised mentally yet my brain kept working out what I would do when I came out. I never doubted that I would be discharged, and I planned ahead. Music was my secret weapon against loneliness and against people saying cruel or negative things about my lack of progress.

It had taken ten months for me to lift my right foot one inch above the bed sheet. The physiotherapists had given up on me. No rehabilitation program was considered worthwhile. I would spend my life in a wheelchair. Why waste time on me?

In the forty-bed geriatric ward — the lot of long-term patients — we had a four-hourly bedpan round, and bad luck if you wet the bed (or worse) in the meantime. Many of us did, and it was time-consuming for the nurses but humiliating for us.

Because I was regarded as a waste of time, in that the staff were busy and others were easier to rehabilitate, I had all the more reason to do something for myself. In a way this was better, because self-motivation is often more powerful than being forced to do things in some pre-planned program. It made me proud of what I was going to achieve. I was going to bring up my baby, make my husband happy, learn to walk and make a contribution to society in some way.

I had the same idea about returning home. Keep on fighting, I told myself. Little did I know how hard that would be. Due to hospital regulations my baby had not been allowed to visit at all. Being separated from my adored boy until he was nearly two was unbearable, but his beautiful picture by my bedside urged me on. I wanted so much to hold him in my arms, to walk with him. No one else believed in me, only I did.

How lucky I was to have someone, something, to live for, and that aim — getting well for my husband and baby — was my mantra. I was not going to be a kind of doomed Madame Butterfly, committing suicide (not trying to walk) or giving up my baby. The parallel with the operatic story that I knew so well was to become a part of my life which I never could have foreseen.

On my first night home my husband announced he was in love with another woman and that she was pregnant by him, the baby due in three months' time. Horrified and stunned, I told him to leave right away, not to hang around out of pity. Yes, he could see our baby whenever he wanted to. He went. He had put Philip in his cot and waited for him to go to sleep before getting up his courage to give me the news he had withheld on his daily visits, visits lasting only thirty minutes, as permitted under the hospital regulations of the time.

Using the wheelchair carefully as a frame, I leaned into the cot, over my sleeping baby, embraced him and fell asleep thus, weeping. (That scene from *Madame Butterfly* flew into my mind:

at least, unlike Cio-Cio-San, I was keeping my baby and my husband's new love was not going to take him away from me.) Later, when I awoke, I put myself to bed, crawling to the bathroom, too exhausted by grief to make decisions about how I was to cope. I had no support network, no relatives I could call on. It was a 'challenging' time.

Pain was an immense and constant presence. When I was in hospital, how much I had hung out for yet another injection of what sounded like 'pethilorphan', which was administered four-hourly, as an addition to the morphine drip in my arm. Relief lasted a mere ninety minutes then my countdown in and out of hell would begin. (Nowadays, patients are given a self-controlled device in a drip, which gives them a dose of morphine when they need it. The dose is small and more constant so the awful see-saw of pain control I experienced is not such an issue.)

After the first six weeks, the pain lessened slightly and I was given only aspirin, a sudden withdrawal eased only by barbiturates for sleep. The doctors feared I might get addicted to stronger opiates (see pages 197–203). Desperately in pain, there was little relief other than the barbiturates, so I was dosed heavily and slept away much of the day. When I was discharged, I was given a bottle of barbiturates. I poured them down the toilet immediately after my husband left. They were no use to me. I had a baby who might wake and need my assistance. I had to learn independence and that was all that mattered.

Fortunately, and I have always found good fortune and inspiring people around me, neighbours rallied and new friends appeared. After six months I had learned to use Philip's pram as a walking frame and extended my walking from around our flat in Abingdon to the outside — to the washing line, to the corner shop, and eventually to the village one whole English mile away.

My pain was controlled with paracetamol alone. Many tears were shed. But somehow, with beautiful young Philip beside me, crawling at first and then helping me learn to walk — playing opposite roles, with him as leader — I made it. My exercises were those I remembered from ballet lessons as an under-five. Who could ever have thought the importance of those lessons at the time? Gradually, I did my own program of physiotherapy.

Friends strengthened my resolve towards independence. I gained a scholarship to a teacher training college in nearby Oxford. A car was necessary because, although I had given the wheelchair back to the hospital as soon as I could, I still limped and could not walk far. I purchased the car on the never-never, as we called it then, and undertook my three years of professional training.

Through all this, the staff of the clinic and of the hospital where I had worked as a research assistant before the accident kept in touch, visited, helped and encouraged me. Now that I had to support my son, they gave me work in the academic vacations so I could earn extra money, because my scholarship, a mere ten pounds per week, was barely adequate. How lucky I was having work and a professional life to fall back on, not just for financial aid but as a social network — this was a way of dealing with pain by distraction. Hospital staff looked after Philip while I worked as a research assistant again after I qualified as a teacher, and then, six years after the accident, I was accepted as a migrant back to

Australia, a country I loved and where I had spent most of my pre-teenage years.

All this led me to Sydney and the field of teaching children with physical and emotional difficulties. For many years I worked with children suffering from varying degrees of disability. Then, after further years working in opera, coaching singers in foreign languages, and for television, it seemed only natural to go back to teaching, albeit in a part-time capacity.

Living with chronic pain is a great teacher, and I hope I have gained an understanding of the suffering of others. It's been forty-five tough years for me, with many setbacks, the kind that all people in chronic pain probably encounter.

There have been fifteen further attempts to correct my spinal and pelvic injuries. In 1992 I had a setback that made me accept a wheelchair once more. But I am one of the lucky ones. The doctors' prognosis was wrong. I can walk, at least a little. To someone who is unable to walk one step, walking 100 metres is like climbing Everest. So to all of you I say: have courage and confidence in yourself. To the French novelist Honoré de Balzac (1799–1850), it was important that one 'should write not of himself but about the pain of others, not that which one sees in the mirror.' My pain is your pain, we understand one another.

I offer this book as a grain of sand in your ocean of discovery and I hope it will be of some help to some of you some of the time.

1

Pain Explained

What does 'pain' mean? You can speak of emotional and psychological pain, or think of any type of suffering as a kind of pain, but I want to start with the plain and simple one, physical pain. 'It hurts, stupid!', as a sensible child told me. Of course, physical pain involves emotional and psychological suffering as well, and I have much to say about this too.

It helps to have some idea how physical pain is caused. There are two good reasons for looking at the 'how it works' of pain. One is so that you can better understand the language your doctor and other health professionals use when they are talking about pain — because they may have a very different understanding from you, based on their technical training. Good, free and fearless communication is very important in being able to cope with pain, and it certainly helps if you and your doctor/therapist are not talking at cross purposes.

And knowing how pain 'works' makes it easier to understand how treatments work. This may help you to have realistic expectations and to use treatments effectively. Also it might make it easier for you to make informed choices about the treatments offered to you, including some less 'mainstream' treatments, which may not always offer good value for money or time.

Types of pain

Pain can be classified in various ways. It is like cutting up a cake in different ways: slices, wedges or chunks. Each way of dividing it is interesting and useful in its way, but it remains the same cake.

One such division is pricking, burning or aching pain. Each of us will recognise these from our own experiences. Different types of nerve fibres seem to be responsible for carrying the message of these different qualities of pain, and these qualities may help a doctor make a diagnosis about what kind of problem is going on.

Another way of dividing pain is into 'acute' and 'chronic'. Again, it is helpful to know what doctors and other health professionals mean when they use these words. A lot of us use 'acute' to mean *really* bad and chronic to mean really *bad*. But health professionals mean something quite specific when they use these words. Acute pain is of short duration — like the pain of a heart attack or appendicitis, a kidney stone or an attack of gout. Chronic pain is of longer, more continuous duration — like the pain of osteoarthritis.

Another important factor is the severity of pain. Nowadays it is common to use a simple scale to describe levels of pain. It generally goes from one to ten, with one being the least severe and ten the most unbearable. A doctor might ask, 'How bad is your pain on a scale of one to ten, when one is quite bearable and ten is really extremely bad?' This is not very scientific, but it is surprisingly useful, especially for measuring changes in your pain level. It is less useful for comparing different people's pain, of course, since everyone is different.

Why do we have pain?

A biologist will answer this question pretty simply: pain is protective. It gives a warning of harm and tells the organism to beat a hasty retreat.

Let's imagine that a creature comes into contact with a very hot saucepan or something nastily sharp like a cat's claw. What happens is that the ends of certain nerves of the body, called pain fibres, detect the tissue damage and send a message back to the nerve centre of the body. Even in primitive creatures with no brains, this is instantly linked up with a signal to certain muscles to 'Get the hell out of there!' This is called a 'withdrawal reflex' and is what you experience when you accidentally touch something like the hot saucepan — your muscles have acted well, possibly before you have become aware of the pain, and certainly before you have time to think about it.

The withdrawal reflex is important because if the pain continues in a low-grade fashion it causes muscle spasm, which is itself painful and can make your pain a lot worse. The withdrawal reflex is important in understanding some sorts of pain and some things you can do about it.

Creatures with no brains have these sorts of reflexes. But can we say they experience pain if they never become aware of it? Most of us don't think twice about boiling up shellfish. But what about fish, which do have brains? Most people are happy enough to accept that catching a fish is OK, arguing that, although its body might be experiencing pain, the fish has no consciousness — something that others might dispute. However, most people would agree that sheep, rabbits, dogs, horses and other mammals do experience pain and accept that it is our responsibility to minimise that pain.

As for humans, we not only have awareness of pain but we think about our pain too. If that means our suffering is greater than that of the fish, it also means we can influence our pain with the ways we think and act.

Pain and the human nervous system

Obviously our nervous system is more complex than that of a mollusc's. It is not necessary to understand all its complexities, but a few concepts help.

Pain fibres from all parts of the body connect to the spinal cord, which is a thick bundle of nerve fibres (rather like telephone cables) known as the central nervous system. Don't get confused here. The spinal *cord* runs in a canal protected by the bones of the spine: the spine and spinal cord are not the same thing.

Pain fibres are nerve fibres and they have a direct connection with other nerve fibres running back to the muscles. When you experience pain, the circuit of nerve fibres connected to the muscles in the part of the body where the pain came from produces the withdrawal reflex.

In the spinal cord, there are also connections with other types of nerve fibres: with 'touch' fibres, for instance, which tell you when something is touching or pressing on you, and with fibres that indicate the position of your joints or the length of your muscles.

Interestingly, if enough 'noise' is coming from these other sources, it can reduce the signals relayed from the pain fibres up the spinal cord. This is known as 'gating'. Think of a porter at the gate (or someone at the window) who closes it when there is a lot of noise outside, and you are getting close to the idea of gating. Gating is a useful model for understanding several of the treatments for chronic pain; for example, it may explain the benefits of TENS machines, acupuncture, 'deep heat' and even rubbing your arm when you hit your funny bone.

The spinal cord has to coordinate a whole lot of different messages — after all, it is not much use your arm muscles withdrawing from a hot saucepan if your hand muscles are doing the opposite. Pain from one part of the body also has effects on other parts of the body, with messages going up and down the spinal cord via 'relay' nerves. Don't be surprised when pain in one part of your body has effects on other parts, especially in adjacent parts: every osteopath knows that a problem in the neck can cause a pain in the jaw (although your doctor may be less likely to accept the idea).

At the very top of the spinal cord sits the brain, which has 'primitive' parts (like a fish brain has) and also the clever bits that make us aware and give us the ability to think. Pain fibres have two important relay connections in the more primitive parts, and these are important in the 'fight or flight' response of the body: if something causes you pain, your body is programmed to fight it or run.

One important connection is in that part of the brain that regulates how awake or 'aroused' we are. This makes sense because getting away from a painful burn or cat scratch is a lot harder if you are still asleep. But there is a downside. If you are constantly aroused by chronic pain, causing sleep disturbance (insomnia), this can make your pain worse. It's important to be aware that this arousal may be going on at the subconscious level of the brain, especially when you have chronic pain.

Another primitive part of the brain coordinates the function of our internal organs. Responding to a painful cat scratch is easier if your heart is pumping thirteen to the dozen, your breathing is fast and if certain interesting things happen to your intestines. But this bodily experience of anxiety can make the pain worse, especially when it increases muscle tension in the body. Pain causes anxiety symptoms, and these can worsen pain. Such anxiety is not about being neurotic, it's physical. It is part and parcel of the experience of pain, and it is important for doctors and patients alike to recognise and accept it.

Finally, in the 'higher' parts of the brain, there are relay connections of pain fibres which give us our awareness of pain, help us to interpret it, decide on action and integrate the pain with our emotional responses.

The pain threshold

You might hear talk about the pain 'threshold', which is the point at which a person experiences pain — for example, how sharp a knife has to be before it causes you to feel pain. At first, you might think this is very different from one person to another — after all, some people and some cultures, such as the unflinching Native Americans, are known to be especially stoic about pain. In fact, pain thresholds don't vary all that much between different people, and they certainly don't vary systematically between cultures, yet the way people experience pain obviously does vary a great deal. The power of the brain to alter our experience of pain is shown by the way some people can endure pain in special circumstances, such as walking on hot coals.

Our experience of pain is influenced by our emotions, by our expectations and fears, and especially by what we have learned in our previous experiences of pain. So if your doctor talks about these things, don't be offended by the idea that it is all in your head, because in fact all pains are experienced through the mind.

The good news is that this gives us another avenue of modifying or controlling our pain.

Causes of pain

What sorts of things can set pain fibres firing off messages to the nerve centres of the body? The typical situation is when some thing or other irritates the nerve endings. This is usually a chemical released by injury, whether the injury be a burn, physical trauma or some kind of disease. Doctors generally use the word 'trauma' to mean a physical injury, whereas most of us think of trauma as anything particularly shocking — another example of how language can lead to misunderstandings.

Inflammation

When doctors talk about 'inflammation', patients may have only a vague idea of what they mean. Many types of pain happen through a process of inflammation. Inflammation is the body's response to any of a number of damaging 'insults', whether it be a poison (such as alcohol), an injury (like a sprained ankle) or a virus in the stomach.

Most of us know what sunburn feels and looks like. We know the skin gets red and hot and may get visibly swollen, especially if there are blisters. And it hurts.

Here are the four signs of inflammation: redness, swelling, heat and pain. '*Rubor, tumor, calor, dolor*' goes the chant in Latin (nowadays your doctor will not speak Latin to impress you and to keep you in the dark, like doctors used to do).

The body reacts to an injury with a rush of blood to the area (causing redness and heat) and the release of lots of fluids. The fluids, which cause swelling, contain white blood cells and all sorts of enzymes to fight off any foreign bodies and to promote healing. Healing often involves producing some 'scar tissue', which is a kind of generic all-purpose tissue — think of it as being like Polyfilla used for repairing cracks in buildings.

Now we come to the most important point of this section. Those enzymes and chemicals in the inflammatory fluid powerfully stimulate pain fibres, causing *acute* pain. If this process persists it will cause *chronic* pain. Even old scar tissue can cause chronic pain if it presses on nerves or upsets the orderly function of muscles, joints and ligaments.

To make it easier to understand your doctor, it is good to know that any word with '-itis' on the end just means inflammation of that particular part of the body. Hepatitis is inflammation of the liver, sinusitis is inflammation of the sinus, gastroenteritis is inflammation of the stomach and intestines, dermatitis is inflammation of the skin, arthritis is inflammation of the joints. There are dozens of such examples.

Two important causes of inflammation are infections and autoimmune diseases, but other things, such as poisons, can also cause inflammation. Alcohol is poison which like other poisons used in low doses (such as arsenic) can possibly even be relatively beneficial. It is, however, a toxin that, in excess, causes myocarditis, gastritis, cardiomyopathy, colitis, proctitis and hepatitis.

Although inflammation is a protective process, it may give us pain signals that we don't really want or need. There is a whole series of 'anti-inflammatory' medicines that are used to reduce pain and other symptoms of inflammation, ranging from aspirin through to the recently controversial Vioxx.

Infection and inflammation

The most common cause of inflammation is infection, whether it be the 'flu, food poisoning, a tooth abscess or a urinary tract infection. But not all inflammation is caused by an infection. For example, although arthritis can be caused by an infection (so-called 'septic arthritis'), it is more often the result of wear and tear ('osteoarthritis') or of autoimmune disease ('rheumatoid arthritis').

Autoimmune disease

A substantial number of people, including children, with chronic pain have some sort of autoimmune disease. 'Autoimmune' means that, instead of attacking foreign bodies like bacteria, the immune system gets muddled and attacks some part of the body itself. Rheumatoid arthritis is perhaps the best known case. When the immune system acts this way, it causes inflammation and may eventually cause scarring. Both of these can cause pain.

For autoimmune disease, medicines such as cortisone used particularly in joint injections or orally may be needed to damp down the unhelpful immune activity.

Oxygen, muscle spasm and pain

There are two other special related cases when chemicals in the body can make pain fibres go haywire, and both happen when a part of the body is starved of oxygen. All parts of the body need oxygen, carried by the blood, to keep functioning. The muscles of the body, especially, do not take kindly to being deprived of oxygen. In fact, when there is not enough oxygen, muscles begin to hurt like hell. This is probably because they switch over to an emergency energy supply that produces lactic acid, a chemical that fires off pain fibres.

There is a well-known dramatic example of this. The 'mother of all muscles' is the heart. When the heart runs short of oxygen, usually because of coronary artery disease, it causes the pain known as 'angina' and, if this persists, the pain of an actual heart attack. Doctors call this 'ischaemic' pain, which means pain from lack of blood supply. Angina is a type of acute ischaemic pain, but it is usually recurrent — that is, it tends to occur again and again (but not continuously, so is not chronic pain).

Other muscles of the body can suffer from lack of oxygen. For instance, a muscle cramp occurs when a muscle that runs out of oxygen goes into spasm, produces lactic acid and causes acute pain. Runners and swimmers know the risk of cramps all too well, and they know not to exercise after eating because this is a time when the body moves its oxygen-rich blood supply to the intestines to help absorb food.

We can begin to put these ideas together. Imagine a chronic pain that causes a chronic withdrawal reflex in muscles — the muscles are in low-grade spasm — and the result is a spreading and worsening of the original pain.

For the person with chronic pain, from whatever source, this is a danger to be reckoned with. Have a look at a picture of the muscles of the human body and see just how many muscles there are, both great and small. Any single one of them can cause severe pain if it goes into spasm, and also more subtle pain and insidious pain that might even defy your doctor's diagnostic powers.

Muscle spasm is a protective reflex that may give us unhelpful pain. Many treatments, including medicines like diazepam (Valium), are used to reduce pain caused by muscle spasm.

Neuropathic pain

Neuropathic pain is another term doctors use. This type of pain does not start at the nerve ending that is detecting tissue damage, but in the nerve fibres that send messages to the spinal cord, up the spinal cord and to various parts of the brain. When there is neuropathic pain, these nerve fibres are firing out of control. Think of it this way: the message is not coming from the telephone receiver, but from a malfunction somewhere in the telephone cables or telephone exchange.

This pain can happen in several different ways. One is when something presses on a nerve, as often happens in people who have problems of the spine: nerves are particularly vulnerable to pressure where they pass through narrow windows in the spine to enter and leave the spinal cord.

Another case is when the nerve is injured by a poison or disease: alcoholics and untreated diabetics can get nerve damage causing chronic neuropathic pain. Viruses can also injure nerves and cause neuropathic pain, like 'trigeminal neuralgia' (which is a neuropathic pain in the trigeminal nerve, in the face).

One of the most telling examples is 'phantom pain', when a person feels pain in a limb that has been amputated: clearly the nerves which used to represent that part of the body are sending wrong, and unhelpful, messages.

Neuropathic pain often does not respond well to the usual types of painkillers. It can be treated with medicines that damp down the firing of the nerves and are more commonly used to treat depression and epilepsy.

Referred pain

This just means that a pain is experienced not where you might expect it to be. Most of us, knowing the heart is usually on the left side of the chest, would expect this to be where heart pain is felt, but actually there is a medical rule of thumb that pain over the heart is often not coming from the heart.

There is no need for us to go into the reasons for this — it is up to doctors to make accurate diagnoses. The important thing for us as patients is to remember that the source of a pain may not always be what we think it is. Common examples are when people have a pain under the right ribs, which they think is from their liver because that is where the liver is; and when people have a pain in the flanks which they are convinced is coming from their kidneys. In these cases the pain is very often coming from the muscles and ligaments of the spine.

2

Dealing with Health Professionals

The choice of a good doctor can mean the difference between you dreading and delaying each visit and a relaxed relationship conducive to your health. In the UK and in France we are fortunate to have a choice of doctors, unless we live in an isolated country area — in which case we are lucky to have a doctor at all. In the metropolitan area of most cities there are sufficient doctors for the population, although it may happen that the best or most popular ones are heavily booked.

You should play your role in establishing this important relationship just as much as the doctor must. Let's imagine the situation when you are sick and are visiting a new doctor for the first time. If your condition is a complex one, it would be wise to book a long consultation, both to be practical and as a courtesy to the doctor and other patients in the waiting room. It is helpful to write down the reasons for your visit before you go, and make a copy of your notes for yourself as well as one for the doctor. When we are unwell we do not always think clearly, so it is a good idea to have notes to refer to, particularly if you are nervous or find it difficult to explain your past medical history.

It works well to have a list noting symptoms such as:

- severe headache
- nausea
- difficulty sleeping
- pains in the abdomen.

Keep the list to a manageable size, with five points at most. Believe it or not, at one surgery I saw a notice stating: 'Due to pressure of the doctor's time, patients are urged to complain of only one symptom per visit.' Imagine a dangerously sick asthmatic who has broken his foot in a bike accident and is frightened to mention both ailments. I am happy to say the notice was not there long.

Doctors and nurses distinguish between 'symptoms' and 'signs'. It helps to know the difference so you can understand them. *Symptoms* are things a person complains of: for example, a pain or a cough, nausea or vomiting, dizziness or numbness. *Signs* are things the doctor finds when she examines you, like an irregular pulse, an enlarged liver, a high temperature.

Some things can be both a symptom and a sign. A person may complain of jaundice (yellow eyes and skin), for instance, and the doctor may observe it. But some things — including pain — are only ever symptoms and the doctor cannot see them (although a patient writhing about is a clear sign of pain). Pain is a symptom, but tenderness when the doctor presses your belly is a sign; likewise, an itch is a symptom, but scratch marks are signs.

It is useful to make a succinct summary of your complete medical history in chronological point form. This can save a doctor lots of time and leave time for talking about the important things. I always take one if I see a new doctor, and I produced one for my child years ago. Now he is grown up, it is a useful reference for him when he goes overseas. Include in it a list of any medications to which you are allergic or intolerant (and the type of reactions you experienced).

Below is an example of the sort of medical history that will be helpful to your doctor.

Medical history: Jennifer Dickson (b. 13/09/1939)

1945 Tonsillectomy

1952 Sinus operation to correct blockage

1956 Appendectomy

1973 Viral encephalitis

1983 Viral pericarditis [a viral infection of the pericardium, the membrane covering the outside of the heart]

1989 Cervical laminectomy

2004 Total left hip replacement

Allergies and drug sensitivities: Penicillin (swollen face), Maxolon & Stemetil (lockjaw).

Current medication: MSContin 40 mgs daily; diazepam 5–10 mgs at night; paracetamol as required.

At the appointment, allow the doctor time to consider your symptoms and wait to be examined. Your blood pressure might be measured. If you are concerned about this don't be afraid to ask; if you don't know what the normal reading should be for your age, ask that too. Many doctors assume that we understand or that we don't need to know. I like to know: it's my body after all.

Establishing that you care about your condition does not show that you are a hypochondriac. Your doctor will find it easier to care for you if you explain carefully what you expect and/or think that you need. On the other hand, we can't go in and instruct the doctor how to do the job — it sets the relationship off on a very poor footing. This is a delicate area and it is worth thinking about the doctor's perspective. He or she may have had experience of suspicious or thorny patients who have read just enough to make them dangerous. This presents a challenge for the doctor of course — but the patient should try to imagine what it is like sitting in the other chair.

Some patients demand much more information than others, and some really prefer to believe the 'doctor knows best'. Both positions are valid. One problem with wanting lots of explanation and information is that the doctor may be under huge time pressures — so it is always good to remember those who are still sitting in the waiting room. Most doctors will be grateful if a patient suggests coming back at another time to talk over some things in more detail if necessary. Keeping a few notes is a good idea — after all, the doctor should keep notes too. If the doctor is really uncomfortable with explaining things in detail (and, let's face it, some are, either because they are a bit unsure or insecure themselves, or too busy, or a bit old-fashioned, or feel threatened by patients wanting to know a lot), then you might need a different doctor.

If you do choose a doctor whom you subsequently do not like or who seems to have taken a dislike to you, don't be afraid to change. If you move to another practice you can ask and offer to pay for copies of your previous records if you have had many consultations. These, or more likely a summary of them with copies of important reports and correspondence, will be sent to your new doctor once you advise details; it is not normal practice for these to be sent to the patient. There is an understandable reluctance on the part of some practitioners to allow us to see what they have written about us, and sometimes this is just as well.

These days we have to be mindful of the cost factor in consultations and grateful when our practitioners give us good care. However, the doctor is quite entitled to charge for the work involved in preparing this paperwork, which may be considerable. After all, a lawyer would not prepare summaries and copies of documents for free.

I recommend you go to your consultation smartly dressed. A dear friend pointed out that it is harder for people to be nasty to her if she is well dressed. Although this may be pure imagination, it works for her. Certainly dressing in clean, neat clothes is a form of politeness, of status, of putting your best side forward. And it is good to do this when you are feeling insecure and uncertain of yourself. Many people reject this notion as being selective or politically incorrect. Make whatever choice you wish, of course. These are only suggestions.

If you are taking your child for a consultation, much the same advice will apply, but allow the child, depending on his age, to speak for himself.

Admission to hospital

On admission to hospital, if it is appropriate or possible, make sure you give details of past medical history. If yours is a complicated story, it's a simple task to write it out when you are well in order to have it ready for emergencies.

Keep it safe in a place you can easily find, such as with your passport or travel documents, somewhere your family can find it without wasting important time. Increasingly, GPs keep compu-terised records. It's a good idea to request a copy of test results and correspondence they have on record about you. Not only is it in your best interests but there could be errors, either because you gave your history at a time you were stressed, or someone made an error in transcribing from the doctor's notes.

When we are suffering from acute pain it's really difficult to recall all the details and medications that are essential for the treating medical team to know.

If you are allergic to certain medicines, it is important that you have this written down and that you carry this list with you in your wallet, briefcase or handbag. Penicillin is one drug that is given in error and can have catastrophic side effects. It is much simpler to have information at the ready than to cause a tragedy by neglecting to remember. Some people with significant health risks choose to buy a medi-alert badge or bracelet, a device on which such details are noted. They are available from most large pharmacies.

If you are sensitive to certain drugs, you may be asked to describe the symptoms you suffered — for example, with penicillin it may have been huge hives or a significant rash, other drugs cause facial contortions or may induce vomiting and nausea.

Careful use of language

In using language, particularly with children, it is important to be careful of the pictures we paint. Here are some examples that are self-explanatory and obviously best avoided.

- 'Don't worry about your operation, the doctor will knock you out.'
- 'The doctor will put you to sleep' (but the cat was put to sleep recently by the vet).
- 'Doctor will give you a nice needle and you won't feel a thing' (nice and needle are not words that go together for most of us).

The same can apply to everyday terms. The word 'drug' has some negative associations due to illicit uses, whether prescription or illegal. So it may be useful to refer to medicines as medication or tablets (or spray, syrup, even injections), or some doctors prefer to use the word 'medicines'.

We have become oversensitive to certain words and no longer use simple terminology. An elderly blind friend of mine, aged ninety-two, hates being referred to as 'visually impaired'. As she argues, 'visually impaired' could mean that she needs strong glasses, whereas if you say she is blind, people know she simply cannot see. It seems ridiculous not to use terms that people who suffer from disabilities themselves regard as perfectly acceptable.

Wheelchair patients are also referred to in many strange ways, such as 'mobility challenged'. I am happy to be plonked under the category of 'wheelie' myself, a good local expression that indicates I use a wheelchair. If, on the other hand, someone says I am mobility challenged, does it mean I limp, am an amputee, that I walk with a strange gait, or that my arthritis slows me down?

Likewise, if somebody is stone deaf, they may prefer people to understand they cannot hear rather than to think they are just missing the occasional word. To be 'hard of hearing', the old phrase, is more sensible than 'sound challenged'.

Finding the right words

Using the right language to express what you mean is especially important for children and young people, who are very susceptible to the opinions of their peers (see Suzy's story, pages 149–54). Children must be helped to understand that medication prescribed by doctors has a therapeutic use and is intended to make them better. Under no circumstances must young people be made to feel that being unwell is something weird which alienates them from their peers. Nor must they feel ashamed that they require tablets or pills.

Language can encourage a child to display fortitude and strength when injured — for example, if she falls and breaks her wrist and is naturally preoccupied with that, ask her, 'How's your other wrist?' By changing her focus, she may lose concentration on the sore wrist and examine the good one. Likewise, a child frightened by the sight of his own blood may be greatly cheered if you congratulate him by saying, 'Wow, that *is* a fantastic colour. You know, that blood shows your body is doing its work trying to heal the wound, and the flow of blood is actually cleaning the wound as it comes out.'

By changing the notion of a word you can take its power away — for example, many therapists now refer to 'discomfort' instead of pain. They also seem to find that speaking of tumours rather than a cancer is less frightening. If a child has several 'attacks' of pain, it might be better to call it an 'episode'. Children themselves can be good at adapting language with each other.

Reassurance is important too. 'Honey, I know your arm hurts from your fall, but look at the way that dog in the park is jumping. Isn't he beautiful?' That combines distraction with reassurance. 'I know the wound hurts badly at the moment, but won't it be good when it is better? And it will be better soon.' The word 'soon' seems to work wonders, as it is one relatively free of fearful connotation — vague yet hopeful.

Not only patients and parents, but doctors and other health professionals need to consider the effect of their words. 'What have you done to yourself?' asked the practice managing doctor who had never seen me at a consultation before and hadn't bothered to read my well-organised and complete but brief notes on the computer in front of him. At that time I had been attending the country practice for four years, on crutches or in a wheelchair, so seeing me standing on crutches should not have provoked such a question. There is a chance that he was attempting banter, but it was offensive. Of course you can learn to laugh, as I did, explaining the situation, and why I was there for my fortnightly review, as required for my morphine prescription reassessment.

A second opinion

Using some of the ideas above (making notes, having an agenda), your interview with a consultant will become more useful. Gone are the days when we were forced to view our medical practitioners as some sort of gods before whom we cowered in fear lest we ask the wrong question. Right up until the 1970s, most people would not have dared to ask a doctor anything, and I know many who are now in their sixties and seventies who would never ever question anything 'the doctor said'.

In these more enlightened times, doctors are used to being approached and being approachable. Most welcome questions and your active involvement in treatment alternatives. It makes their work easier if they feel you understand what is going on.

Once you have dispensed with the formalities and pleasantries, ask your questions, indicate you want to know what will happen in the natural course of events, how treatment may affect this and what risks are involved. Be forthright, and keep it as simple as you can. This will set the tone of the consultation: it should be comforting to understand that the preferred medical model these days is the 'shared' decision model.

Before you go to the consultation, if a serious illness is the likely diagnosis, discuss with your family support group or partner whether or not you want one of them with you. If the sick person is a child, decide whether or not he should be in the room throughout the consultation. This will depend on sensitivity as well as on age; if in doubt, discuss this with the doctor in private.

If you learn that you, your partner or your child has a serious illness, you will probably want to ask many things, about the treatments available and their side effects, length of stay in hospital, absence from work or school — plus all the issues you have considered prior to consultation. Don't be so shocked that you forget to ask such vital questions. Your prepared list will help here. You need not mince words: say what bothers you and, if you are terrified, say so. If you tend to get nervous, that's fair enough too. Tell the doctor you'd rather know the worst, or whatever it is you want. Learn everything you can from the consultant and then go home and have a good cry if you need to. Or have a cry in front of the consultant if that's how you feel. You shouldn't feel fear or shame about showing a doctor you are afraid. The only bravery awards you need lie within the spirit, which helps you to live life to the fullest once you know what you are dealing with.

If there is bad news — whether cancer or some other serious illness — it is very likely that a consultant rather than your GP will be the one to give you the news.

There is always much that can be done to help the patient, even if it is not to be found within traditional medical science. However, orthodox science-based medicine has many procedures to help treat advanced disease and severe chronic pain, as do complementary therapies.

When insult is added to injury

So far, we have assumed that visiting a medical practitioner is a positive experience. This is not always the case, which is why we must be aware that all doctors do not share the view of kindness, trust, hope and belief in their patient's history. I know parents who burst into tears when recounting their frustration and grief about doctors not considering their very sick child to be in need of hospitalisation.

One mother reported that she took her feverish six-year-old son to the nearest accident and emergency department, knowing from previous experience that he needed to be flown by helicopter to a major city hospital. But she was told to take him home and give him one paracetamol every four hours and then see if he 'settled'. The mother was treated as if she were hysterical and attention seeking, but in fact she knew much more about her son's life-threatening condition than the young registrar could possibly ascertain from a brief physical examination. It was not until she insisted on calling a paediatrician at a major specialist hospital that she was afforded the politeness and treatment that ultimately saved her young son's life (the child was flown by helicopter to the teaching hospital).

Better information would avoid some of the disbelief that people with chronic pain feel. There is a great need for a national register of chronically ill patients, or computerised individual medical records that can be accessed on secure sites, so that vital and often life-saving information can be seen quickly by any treating doctor. This could be very important for people with chronic pain who are seeing a doctor for the first time, who have no medical records available and who are requesting opiate medication (see page 197). There are privacy concerns about keeping a national register, but such a system could be available for people with chronic illnesses, without it being compulsory.

Certain physical conditions have received 'a bad press' and, as a result, the attitudes of some health professionals who treat us have become jaded and untrusting. Common complaints include disbelief that the patient — whether adult or child — is actually suffering pain, especially where supporting evidence cannot be found through traditional testing methods, such as radiology, pathology or endoscopy. Just because you are in pain, this does not mean it can necessarily be proved by tests, however sophisticated the technology is becoming.

'You look fine to me,' a new doctor who has never seen you before may remark, although you feel as if death could truly be imminent and almost wish it were, so gravely ill do you feel and so great is the pain.

Patients presenting with chronic pain arising from musculoskeletal disorders such as repetitive strain injuries (RSI) and fibromyalgia, from gynaecological illnesses such as endometriosis and adenomyosis, and from myalgic encephalomyelitis (also known as chronic fatigue syndrome) are among those who have been made to suffer the humiliation of not being believed. They are treated and dismissed as neurotic, work-shy, seeking compensation or as 'gross hysterics'. This term hysteric (from the Greek for 'womb', and referring to the idea that it was caused by a wandering womb, of all things) is often used in a blatantly sexist way. These issues are further discussed in Chapter Eleven (pages 188–201).

If the very people to whom he turns for help lets him down and 'add insult to injury', this may worsen not only the patient's self-esteem but the condition itself, especially if it goes untreated as a result. Sensitive teenagers, already probably embarrassed at being 'different' if they suffer from any illness, are at even greater risk of harm by being disbelieved than are adults. They may also have less self-confidence to deal with other people's doubts or taunts.

Generally I have been more fortunate. My radiological 'proof' is so obvious: no one can ignore the fact that one-third of my pelvis is missing. When requested, I simply take along my bundle of x-rays — which by now almost requires a trolley. The look on the practitioner's face when I offer my 'holiday pics' tells me a lot. Those who laugh, I warm to; with the others, I cross my fingers.

What do you do if you are not believed? Naturally, ask for a second opinion, request further tests and, if you are not satisfied with the hearing you receive, keep seeking an answer. At this point, the patient may, in despair, seek inappropriate or even base-less 'alternative' therapies (see Chapter Six, pages 73–95).

One approach might be to say, 'Doctor, I get the impression you feel sceptical about the nature and severity of my illness. If this is so, please explain the basis of that.' Polite but firm words can turn a growling lion into a very considerate lamb.

If you are referred for psychiatric treatment by a doctor who doesn't believe in your pain, you may even be made to feel 'crazy' or 'hysterical'. This can add enormously to the stress involved in experiencing pain. And doubting yourself can hardly help you have the strength to deal with the pain itself. Psychologists or psychiatrists have an important role in pain management and are better involved as part of the routine, rather than at the end when all else has failed.

Very occasionally people do present themselves with fictitious pain in order to get medical treatment, especially surgery to remove parts of their body. One of the names for this is Munchausen's syndrome. Similarly, very rarely parents present their children as ill when they are not; this is called Munchausen's syndrome by proxy.

There are good and bad reasons for referring people with chronic pain to psychiatrists. Depression is foremost among them — but remember the depression may or may not be caused by the pain. Certainly depression makes it harder to cope with pain, and treating any depression may help people with their pain. People in pain who suffer from chronic anxiety may also benefit from referral to psychiatrists or psychologists. Also, as discussed later, antidepressants can be useful in treating pain in people without depression (see page 57) and sometimes a psychiatrist can be involved here. The danger is when it is implied that a person's complaint of pain is entirely caused by depression or anxiety, which is rarely credible. It is worth pointing out that the social consequences of pain — such as isolation, financial loss and inability to work — may cause more depression and anxiety than the pain itself.

Hopefully, a doctor referring you to a psychologist or psychiatrist will explain the reasons in such a way that you don't feel slighted or disbelieved.

If you have seen several specialists who all agree on a diagnosis and/or prognosis, there comes a time when you just have to accept it graciously, even if it doesn't fit your beliefs or expectations. That does not mean you have to give up hope. It may still be constructive to read about how a condition generally progresses and discover what you can do to make the most of your future life. Doctors can be wrong, like mine were when they proclaimed I would never walk again. In accepting bad news, it is best to set up strategies of small achievable objectives in order to restore optimism.

Factors in healing are not always within the realms of medical science. People of many faiths find strength and courage through praying to a higher power for the best outcome, if not necessarily for cure. I wouldn't presume to judge anybody else's beliefs, and I personally believe that hope, wherever it comes from, is incredibly powerful. Recent medical 'trials' of prayer show no benefit for people with illness, but these prayer sessions have been impersonal; perhaps personal prayer could have some benefit. Some research suggests that those with a religious or spiritual faith do fare better than those who make no acknowledgement of a 'higher power'. We should try not to make assumptions about what people believe.

Probably fewer people with chronic pain are neglected and ignored by medical professionals in western societies now than they used to be, although there are many who miss out. In many countries with public health systems, the best care may not be available to all, given its increasing cost.

Worldwide, more and more litigation is taking place, which at best is a double-edged sword. In some situations, it may be appropriate to take legal action, especially if this is necessary to ensure that you receive appropriate treatment. Yet this may come at a great personal cost. Litigation is stressful and the bitterness and resentment — the 'siege mentality' — that it engenders may be unhelpful to your best health. The same can be true of claims for workers' compensation or other insurance claims. None of this applies in New Zealand, for example: with its no-fault compensation system, health practitioners cannot be sued.

If you are one of those people who have struggled to be believed, it is important that you are able to decide at what point it is better to move on, change your focus away from blaming the system that failed you and concentrate on finding your own solution. There may be many outlets and practitioners available who will offer help and a whole new life, who will reconsider your problem afresh, perhaps more supportively and holistically.

Procedural pain: when your doctor causes pain

A special case of acute pain is when the health professional is the one causing the pain. This is called procedural pain.

Some medical tests, including those required for investigation of pain, are by their nature painful. To acknowledge this is just plain common sense. For example, a lumbar puncture is at best very uncomfortable. If you are anxious about this procedure it may be wise to ask the treating physician to give you a sedative injection in addition to the local anaesthetic (an injection and/or cream), which is applied to the site of the needle puncture (injection). It is difficult to find the correct space in your back for the doctor to withdraw the cerebral spinal fluid, so if she misses this space you will suffer pain as the needle touches other structures. It is usual for children to be given a short low-dose anaesthetic so that they do not experience the pain of this procedure.

In adults, it is expected that we will just grin and bear it. Some of us, however, have endured so many painful treatments that our ability to withstand pain has greatly diminished. Nobody is going to give you a medal for bravery, so if you need pain relief be forthright and ask for it. What a pity we feel so embarrassed to ask for this help, as if it is a favour.

Some people experience acute anxiety when they are in an enclosed MRI facility, especially if they suffer from claustrophobia. MRI stands for magnetic resonance imagery and is a radiological procedure in which parts of the body are scanned via a magnetic device within the machine. You are placed in a capsule, and as the machine scans around your body it makes a loud tapping noise, which frightens some people. You may be sedated to help to calm you, and the radiographer will talk you through the procedure and give instructions, reassurance and enable you to call 'stop' if you become afraid. The trauma to a distressed patient is far greater than the harm of being lightly sedated, unless there are specific clinical indications against it.

If you have very small veins, it may be difficult to extract blood samples and in these cases you might suffer pain also, which is made worse by the frustration of repeated attempts and not knowing whether they will be successful or not. For children, an anaesthetic cream or patch (EMLA, a brand name) can be applied up to ninety minutes prior to the blood test that will require venipuncture. As this cream requires prior planning and time, it is best that the parent ask for it well in advance. Discuss the procedure your child is going to have with the receptionist/nurse and make sure you go to the hospital early, where your child may sit with you in a quiet room, and have the cream or patch applied, allowing it time to work.

After radiological procedures, such as swallowing a 'barium meal', you could become very constipated. Ask the radiographer if the substance you swallowed is likely to give you this reaction and ask for specific advice on stool softeners or laxatives and the correct dosage necessary to rid your body of the substance. Simple precautions, including the use of Sorbolene cream on your toilet paper to soften the anal area, may save you days of stomach-aches and headaches from constipation. If you have a very sore 'tail', use baby oil and cotton wool as a wipe.

3

The Medical Approach

There is a rather arbitrary division between medical and alternative therapies; hence the designation complementary and alternative medicine (or CAM) doesn't necessarily tell us a lot about the quality of the treatments. History demonstrates that yesterday's medical treatment might be tomorrow's quackery and today's alternative treatment might be tomorrow's mainstream.

The pendulum has swung well away from the idea that western medicine has a monopoly on good treatment. It does, however, have the best available processes to reach toward truth, whereas CAM may seem at times to have a different rather 'post-modernist' approach in which truth is what you say it is. Some might ask whether the pendulum has swung too far, where 'anything goes' and all truth is relative.

This issue is very important for people with chronic illnesses, including people with chronic pain for which there is no 'cure', because almost any therapy has the potential to do harm — even if it is only harm to your bank balance. As many people with chronic pain suffer economic privation from their disability, this is far from a trivial matter.

There are two interesting things about mainstream western medical treatments. The first is that they are supposed to be based on evidence, and the second is that they are firmly entrenched in our economies. These two features can come into conflict.

Perhaps the best example of this is in the economic power of pharmaceutical companies, which in size rank near the top of the stock exchange in most countries. A drug company makes money if it can create 'illness' — such as by convincing men and women that they need to take a pill to lose weight.

It is also worth bearing in mind that many health-care professionals are running small- or medium-scale businesses and are trying to make a living for themselves and their families. A dentist may have little financial incentive to find the simplest and cheapest solution to your dental needs and, when all is said and done, surgeons get paid for using their scalpels. This issue is not unique to mainstream treatment, of course: a chiropractor makes a buck out of producing those satisfying clicking and cracking sounds.

Headaches are an interesting case. Not so long ago dentists discovered that severe chronic headaches were often caused by people having uneven bites, grinding their teeth in the night, straining their temporo-mandibular joints (which are located just in front of the ear), and consequently putting their necks out of kilter. They encouraged people to have splints made for their teeth to correct the problem. Meanwhile chiropractors remain certain that headaches are usually caused by problems in the alignment of the spine, which also causes people to have uneven bites. Optometrists would think of headaches in terms of eye problems and psychologists would point to increasing stress in modern life causing tension headaches.

Rather than draw a firm line between medical and alternative therapies, I would like to raise some issues about how you decide whether to try a treatment or not — about the way you consider and weigh up 'evidence'.

Is it fair and reasonable to expect people with chronic health problems to do their own research into the treatments on offer? After all, that is why we have experts and health professionals. How can lay people be expected to sift through mountains of medical research, or judge the claims of advocates of some treatment or other?

I will try to take some of the mystery out of various treatments on offer, so that you are more empowered to make your own informed choices, and give you some hints on dealing with ways of finding reliable information.

A note of caution: study after study shows that the internet contains a great deal of lower grade and biased evidence (not selectively medical or checked by professionals), and therefore the over-anxious patient who seeks information can easily become confused. Be careful what you read. It is not always based on significant research but often on anecdotal evidence with a narrow perspective.

It should be possible to use the same principles to make decisions about all treatments, whether they be 'western' or 'eastern', 'holistic', 'natural', 'scientific', 'complementary' or 'mainstream', although sometimes the yardsticks used may need to be a bit different. Third-party funders such as Medicare and insurers can reasonably choose to go with the evidence provided by proven medical research. But the question should be asked: what is the evidence about both benefit and harm? And you need to keep in mind that all practitioners, even those drawing salaries unrelated to the number of services they provide, will have some emotional and economic stakes in the treatment they are offering, and no one has a monopoly on the truth.

Chance findings and science

So many medicines used to alleviate pain are derived from herbal remedies, some of which have similar bases to aspirin, colchicine and opioids, for example. Do not assume just because something is herbal it is likely to be 'ineffective but harmless'. Or think that because something is developed scientifically, it is basically 'unnatural and wicked'.

Take, for example, two sorts of medicines widely used in the treatment of pain.

We don't know who first found that eating the seeds of the opium poppy was good for relieving pain, and it is very likely that this was discovered independently by different people in different parts of the world at different times. But from the opium poppy are derived the drugs known as the opiates, such as morphine and codeine, which are chemical variations on nature's theme. Are these variations, produced by chemists in laboratories, any more unnatural than those produced by chance by nature?

Often science, or what passed for science at the time, has led to discoveries of natural medicines. Following the theory that in nature an antidote is found near a poison, willow bark, which grows in wet places, was first tried for fevers and agues (pain). Bad science led to the finding of good medicine, and later to the development of the aspirin-like drugs.

Folk wisdom and anecdotal evidence

If enough people over enough time swear that something helps for a medical problem, isn't there likely to be some truth in it? Can't we believe the evidence of our own senses? After all, people were using laudanum, which is tincture of opium, to relieve pain for centuries before anyone ever did any scientific tests on it. If hundreds of millions of Chinese have sworn by the benefits of acupuncture for centuries, there must be some truth in it, mustn't there? And surely all those people wouldn't keep going to chiro-practors if they didn't do any good.

Balanced against this idea — where there is smoke there probably is fire — are the cases of millionaire snake-oil salesmen and charlatan faith healers. A famous trick is to discover someone has one leg shorter than the other, mutter a few prayers, and then show that the legs are now equally long — anyone who knows how to tilt the angle of the pelvis can convincingly 'heal' leg length inequality.

In parts of Europe even today, some doctors are as likely to prescribe vinegar socks and a mustard poultice for a bad cold as to write a prescription for antibiotics. Whereas lots of studies have been done on antibiotics proving their effectiveness, I bet there have been almost no studies on mustard poultices. And yet these traditional remedies may do less harm than the over-prescribing of antibiotics.

This brings us to the question of scientific evidence.

Evidence-based medicine

For better or worse — and when you look at the marvellous advances in the treatments of many once-fatal or debilitating diseases, you would have to say for better — scientific medicine requires treatments to be tested and proved. Often they are first tried in the test tube to see if they do anything at all, and usually medicines are tested on animals before being used by people. Painkillers, for example, are tested for their effects on pain responses in rats. Whether or not you think that is ethical, it does provide real evidence that a medicine is not just snake oil.

Then treatments are trialled in humans before being approved by government regulatory bodies for general use.

The most important part of medical evidence is the 'clinical trial', when a treatment is tried out in something like real-life circumstances. The best trials are 'randomised control trials', in which people are assigned at random into two groups: one does not get the treatment, the other does. An independent group administers the trial, choosing the two groups at random. Patients don't get to choose their own treatments and nor do their doctors or the researchers choose who gets what — otherwise they might end up putting all the easy cases in one group and getting the answers they were looking for: 'See, my wonderful new treatment works.' The people who do not get the treatment are called the control group. Throughout and at the end of the trial, the health of both groups is closely monitored and compared: if the people treated do better than the control group, then you have some evidence that the treatment really works.

However, the effect could be just psychological, through the power of suggestion. Maybe the treated group believed they were going to get better, and so they did. To guard against this, the control groups are usually given a dummy treatment (such as a sugar pill), called a 'placebo'. The placebo should look indistinguishable from the real treatment, so that neither the researchers nor the subjects know who is getting the real and who is getting the placebo treatment. This is what is called a 'randomised double-blind control trial', and is the gold standard of evidence-based medicine.

Doctors are sceptical of treatments that haven't been tested in this way: most new medicines will have survived a few randomised double-blind control trials before being approved by the regulatory agencies. However, some doctors will try old treatments in new situations, or they will experiment with ways of using medicines that are considered safe. Your own doctor may do this to try to help you, but will hopefully keep the principles of evidence in mind and will be familiar with the recommendations of specialists and experts who are very familiar with all the studies and trials that have been done.

When you think about it, it is good that treatments have to pass tough tests before being released on the unsuspecting public, and we should be grateful that the medical profession requires these standards. Hopefully, when your doctor gives you a treatment, she has good reason for thinking it is really safe and effective.

Throwing the baby out with the bathwater

There are a couple of problems with evidence-based medicine. One is that a treatment may be effective but no one has proven that it is and. if we require every treatment to have a randomised double-blind control trial, we might end up throwing out the baby with the bathwater by failing to use treatments that may actually be helpful but are just not proven. This can happen in various ways.

Clinical trials are expensive and are usually carried out or sponsored by pharmaceutical companies that hope to make a profit from the treatment. But who can make a profit out of vinegar socks? It is not as though you can patent the idea. Mustard producers might make a killing if the mustard poultice has a comeback, but realistically they wouldn't invest in that kind of research. So clinical research is likely to be biased towards profit-making treatments. Some treatments never get tested and so only have anecdotal evidence to support them. However, there is increasing research into herbs and other therapies: glucosamine plus chondroitin (for arthritis) is one example of a health food supplement that has been proved in successful trials.

Another problem is that in some instances you cannot do randomised trials because withholding a treatment to the control group may adversely affect their health and is therefore unethical (every trial must be approved by an ethics committee before it can go ahead). Or it may not be possible to give a dummy treatment to a control group. For example, it would be possible to stick a hundred needles at random into a person to provide a placebo treatment for testing the benefits of acupuncture, but I don't think anybody would sign up to be a guinea pig for a study like that. I know I wouldn't. Furthermore, only a particularly bad acupuncturist could really be 'blind' to whether he was giving a placebo or a real treatment.

Similarly, it would be pretty difficult to compare different methods of neck manipulation — and it might even be dangerous. It is not surprising that a recent summary of the evidence base for manipulation of the lower back found no evidence of benefit, despite the fact that many people will tell you their experience of going into the osteopath's scarcely able to walk and walking out pain-free.

Another problem with evidence-based medicine is that it is designed to weed out the effects of the 'placebo'. But if a sugar pill makes people feel better, why not use it?

Some experts believe that the 'real' effect of a treatment is the apparent effect minus any placebo effect: in other words, you shouldn't count the placebo effect. Others argue that the placebo has the power of suggestion and — along with the experience of being cared for, the laying on of hands and belief in the power of magic — is an important and a powerful part of treatment. Alternative practitioners are at an advantage here because they can maximise the placebo or non-specific treatment effect in ways that ethical medical practitioners may not feel able to do.

Where does that leave the pain sufferer?

It is helpful to be aware that your doctor needs to have very high standards of proof before accepting a treatment, and therefore recommending it. If he is sceptical about some alternative remedies, he is probably not just being bloody-minded and blinkered.

As a patient, you may feel the need to try some treatments that might not have passed the rules of evidence-based medicine. However, it is prudent always to bear in mind the drawbacks of unproven treatments, including the financial and physical costs. Just because a therapist really believes in a treatment doesn't mean it is necessarily effective — her view may also be biased if she is making a living out of giving that treatment.

As discussed earlier, your experience of pain is influenced by your emotions, expectations and fears, by the ways you think about pain and by how you organise your life. These are all powerful ways of responding to pain. If you do suffer from pain, what serves you best is being able to harness the power of the mind and spirit without having to line the pockets of too many snake-oil merchants along the way.

4

The Medical Management of Pain

There are various elements to the mainstream medical management of pain: medicines, injections and surgery, physiotherapy and psychological treatments, as well as some treatments that might be classified as alternative or complementary.

In recent years, there has been a growing — and very welcome — trend in the medical management of pain with the establishment of pain clinics, often attached to major hospitals. These clinics have the combined expertise of a multidisciplinary team of specialists. The services they offer patients vary, but may include assessment and management strategies as well as advanced treatment options.

Medicines

Analgesics

The word 'analgesic' refers to medicines that relieve pain without making you unconscious. Although all the medicines discussed here are used in pain relief, the word analgesic is mainly used for the opiates and the anti-inflammatory (and similar) medicines.

Opiates and opioids

These are all the medicines produced primarily from the seeds of the opium poppy (such as morphine, codeine, and heroin) or similar medicines which are synthetic (laboratory-made medicines more or less similar to the opium-based medicines — for example, methadone and fentanyl); the term 'opioids' is correctly used to include the synthetic medicines. The opioids can be used to suppress coughs, to stop diarrhoea and to tranquillise, but their most important use is to reduce pain. They were the first pain-killers used in medicine and were prescribed very freely until the early part of the twentieth century, when a movement led by the USA resulted in their use being restricted (making them 'controlled substances') in most jurisdictions.

Opioids all work on specific receptors in the brain and spinal cord, called the opioid receptors. The body also produces chemicals, such as endorphins, which are released in certain situations (see page 99) and which can affect your mood and your perception of pain by their actions on these opioid receptors.

There are differences among these medicines — in their potency and range of side effects, as well as their duration of action. The effects of morphine, heroin and codeine last for a relatively short time (called a short 'action'), and this is why morphine is often given in slow-release forms. Fentanyl can be given in patch form, and methadone has a very long action and can often be given just once a day.

The opioids are discussed in more detail in Chapter Twelve (pages 197–203); however, the main points to remember about them are:

- they are powerful analgesics
- if you use them for long periods, you may become tolerant of them and so need higher doses to get the same effect
- if you suddenly stop taking them after using them for a long time there may be a withdrawal reaction, so it is best to taper their use rather than stop suddenly
- in overdose they can stop you breathing (that's what happens in heroin overdoses)
- they may have certain side effects, such as mental dullness, dry mouth, nausea and especially constipation.

Because of the side effects and development of tolerance, the opioids are not used lightly. But when they need to be used they should be used without fear or shame, because for most people they are such effective analgesics with proven benefits.

Anti-inflammatory medicines

Aspirin was the first of these medicines to be used on a large scale for analgesia. Its spectacular rise in popularity from the end of the nineteenth century was probably one of the reasons for the fall in over-the-counter sales of opium products.

The *aspirin-like analgesics* include a whole range of substances from Naprosyn, Brufen, and Voltaren through to the newer (and much more expensive) COX-2 inhibitors such as Celebrex and the recently withdrawn Vioxx. The anti-inflammatory analgesics all reduce pain by their effects on the chemicals that trigger off pain receptors so that, unlike the opioids, they are acting mostly at the location of the painful organ or tissue, rather than in the brain (with some central nervous system effects). Because pain-causing chemicals are often released by the process of inflammation and these medicines also act to dampen down the inflammation itself, they are particularly useful for problems such as arthritis and for musculoskeletal pains in general.

Most of these medicines reduce fever too, but they tend to cause upper gastrointestinal (oesophagus, stomach, duodenum) symptoms, inflammation, and even erosions or ulcers. The real advantage of the COX-2 inhibitors is that they do not cause as much stomach (gastric) bleeding as aspirin and the others do. This doesn't mean they are more powerful: they are just generally safer to use from the gastrointestinal viewpoint, especially among older people. (People often talk about a medicine being strong — 'Give me a strong antibiotic, Doctor' — not realising that effective medicines are more like sharp knives than great sledgehammers.)

It is ironic that aspirin is the most toxic of these medicines, and yet it is freely available over the counter. It is seldom recommended for use by children anymore because of a rare but serious reaction called Reye's syndrome which can occur. Do not give aspirin for fever control to children under the age of sixteen without expert medical advice. Be aware that many over-the-counter medications, such as Bonjela for infants who are teething, contain salicylic acid (an aspirin derivative).

As a general rule, if you have an allergic reaction to aspirin you should not take any of the other aspirin-like medicines either. Remember this because your doctor might just forget. You are not the only patient she has to look after.

Paracetamol is an interesting medicine that acts in a similar way to the aspirin-like medicines, but doesn't cause stomach bleeding and has little if any anti-inflammatory side effects. It is the safest of the over-the-counter analgesics for most people. You may have heard that it is bad for the liver but, for the vast majority of people (except for alcoholics, who are a high-risk group for liver problems), that is only true if you have a real overdose, of about twenty or more tablets.

Combination analgesics and caffeine: Caffeine doesn't really fit in here, but it is well known to be good for certain types of headaches, such as migraines and hangovers. This leads to a cautionary tale. Caffeine was one of the ingredients of a number of compound proprietary-brand analgesics such as Bex and Vincent's powders, which were heavily marketed as headache treatments during the 1950s, 1960s and 1970s. Most of them contained aspirin and phenacetin (another aspirin-like medicine). Eventually, many cases of irreversible kidney damage and kidney failure were linked to consumption of large numbers of the powders. Some people had been using up to twenty or thirty doses a day. Caffeine is mildly addictive and, if you are a heavy user, withdrawal causes bad headaches. Many of those who used too many Bex powders were probably getting caffeine-withdrawal headaches if they failed to take the powders: they had become hooked on the very source of their problem. But phenacetin was identified as the major culprit and it is no longer available.

However, the fear about combining one analgesic with another remains, and it is best to consult your doctor before combining medicines like paracetamol or codeine with aspirin-like medicines (Panadeine, Nurofen Plus, Codral).

Cortisone and other steroids are anti-inflammatory substances that are the same as or resemble the steroid hormones produced by the body. They are not classified as analgesics. They may reduce pain by reducing inflammations, such as in acute arthritis. Given in large amounts they can cause dramatic improvement in some inflammatory conditions and they are also used in some cancer treatments. They can be truly life-saving but used long term in moderate or high doses can cause a host of side effects, including weight gain, stomach ulcers, weakening of the bones (osteoporosis) and acne.

It is important not to be scared by horror stories about medicines such as cortisone (the same is true for a lot of medicines with sullied reputations — methadone, for example is excellent for relieving pain as well as for treating heroin addiction). Like all medicines, cortisone-like medicines have benefits to be weighed against side effects. If your doctor suggests or prescribes cortisone-like medicines, it is important to talk over these issues in detail. Local injections of cortisone drugs, when used judiciously as for arthritis, can be very helpful with minimal risks.

Other medicines effective in pain

There are a number of other medicines whose primary use is for different conditions, but which have an important place in the management of pain.

Antidepressants

Antidepressants were developed in the late 1940s and 1950s at a time when the number of medicines available for treating mental illness was increasing rapidly.

As time has gone on, newer antidepressants have been developed and, as is the case with the anti-inflammatory medicines, later generations of antidepressants (especially the Prozac-like group which has been used since the 1990s) have more specific actions and fewer side effects than the old ones. The older antidepressants (the tricyclic agents), however, are still among the most effective available for sleep and pain control. New is not always better.

The antidepressants all work on nerve cells in the brain, changing the balance of the chemicals they use to communicate with other. It is not surprising that they may have effects on other nerves in the body that are important for the transmission of pain signals. They are commonly used for neuropathic pains like trigeminal neuralgia or shingles.

You don't have to be depressed to gain benefit from these medicines: they are often used in lower doses for pain. Low doses may also help alleviate sleep disturbance and anxiety symptoms.

Some people fear becoming addicted to antidepressants, and may have heard horror stories about people getting bad withdrawal reactions when stopping them. It is important to understand that antidepressants are not addictive, but should be tapered slowly rather than stopped abruptly. You can get a bad reaction if you 'jump off' these medicines, just as you can if you suddenly stop taking a blood pressure medication.

Antiepileptics

As with antidepressants, medicines originally used for treating epilepsy have been found to help with pain, especially neuropathic pain. Less commonly, they are helpful with pains from inflammatory problems like arthritis. Because antiepileptics act in some way to 'stabilise' nerve cells so that they don't fire off signals in an uncontrolled fashion, it is not surprising that they also seem to calm down nerves firing off inappropriate pain signals.

Benzodiazepines

These include diazepam (Valium) and other similar drugs, which tranquillise, relax muscles and can put you to sleep. There is a whole range of them: some tranquillise more than cause sleep, others do the opposite; some are long- and some are short-acting. They are usually reserved for brief use in acute situations.

If anxiety and agitation are worsening pain, tranquillisers can be helpful, especially for certain acute pains such as the pain associated with medical procedures.

Valium itself is especially important as a muscle relaxant. Where an osteopath or chiropractor might prefer to manipulate your 'acute crick neck', hospital emergency departments are more likely to send you away with a couple of aspirin and a Valium — and it may work a treat (although not always). Muscle spasm is often a reflex reaction to pain, which can be self-perpetuating (spasm causes pain which causes more spasm), so it is very important to recognise this problem and break the vicious cycle early. Some kinds of pain, such as kidney stones and pain from the uterus, are associated with worsened spasms in muscles in the back. If the pain doesn't go on too long, muscle relaxants are not needed, but for chronic gynaecological pain they may be helpful.

Short-acting benzodiazepines are good for sleep, and for people with chronic pain a good night's sleep often makes the difference between a good day and a 'hell day'.

Unfortunately, as with opioids, you can become tolerant to the effects of benzodiazepines, needing more and more to get to sleep and to get the same feeling of calmness. People can get a nasty withdrawal reaction if they stop them suddenly. But, luckily, tolerance doesn't develop very much to the muscle-relaxing effects of diazepam.

Benzodiazepines have had a bad name as 'mother's little helpers' because in the past they were prescribed too freely and people became dependent on them. However the pendulum should not be allowed to fall too far back away from these useful medicines — again, it is just necessary for patients to be given good information about their benefits and risks. Most of us are capable of being sensible about these things.

Injections and surgery

Injections of local anaesthetic are used of course for many medical and dental procedures. Injections are sometimes also used for chronic pain. Many GPs will inject cortisone-like medicines into or around inflamed joints and ligaments or other structures — for instance, if you have a painful case of 'tennis elbow' or 'clergyman's knee'. Rheumatologists also use these injections for such conditions as rheumatoid arthritis, and pain specialists may use them where they believe nerves are irritated, such as at the point where they pass through the narrow windows in the spine to join the spinal cord. The cortisone dampens down the inflammation that is causing pain and it reduces irritation of the nerve roots. In some cases, injections of toxins may even be used to destroy nerves that are causing intractable pain. However, it often happens that the injection seems a great success, but that the pain doesn't go away long term.

Cortisone-like injections sometimes need to be repeated every few months and it is important to weigh up the risk of weakening the tissues where they are injected over time. In the case of overuse injuries (RSI), some doctors have used cortisone injections, but there is a question whether there is inflammation in these cases; most physiotherapists are very sceptical about injections being used for overuse injuries (see pages 191–96).

Surgery has an important place in certain medical conditions that cause pain. Obviously it is best to take out an appendix or a kidney stone if it is causing pain. Knee and hip replacements are becoming a more common way of dealing with the chronic pain and disability of arthritis, and surgeons obviously do a lot of work patching up those people who are severely injured, as I was.

There are some new and subtle surgical procedures that target irritated or squashed nerves, especially near the spine. (However, nerve cutting is rare these days, as is thermo-coagulation or burning although it is still practised in France.)

Having said that, there are situations in which surgery may be counterproductive, and surgery on the spine often falls into that category. Another case is carpal tunnel operations for overuse injuries of the arm. There are other cases where surgery seems to be indicated but has to be repeated, so that you are left wondering whether it was such a smart idea in the first place.

Prolotherapy is an alternative treatment performed as an adjunct to or instead of steroid injections. Typically, this is an injection that stimulates new tissue growth to tighten and strengthen loose or weak tendons and ligaments, or to repair cartilage in a joint.

Dedicated and ethical doctors will look long and hard at their own results and also keep up with the best advice from experts elsewhere about achieving the best balance of doing good and doing little harm. Yet the surgeon may feel under pressure to operate when nothing else seems to help. As a patient, you are well advised not to put this kind of pressure on surgeons to find a cure for your pain, as it may come back to bite you. It is no dishonour or insult to a doctor to ask for a second opinion. It is hard to undo surgery after it's done, so do remember to get your second opinion before the operation.

Treatment guidelines

In recent years, national health services have published best-practice guidelines for specific diseases. These review international research results for current treatments, in some cases including those for complementary and alternative treatments (see Useful Addresses, page 210).

You should not believe everything you read in the newspapers about medical research. It is easy to clutch at straws when you are in pain, and accept any new miracle story as absolutely true. If a new cure is reported, it is worth checking the reliability of the report and where it was first published. Other things you might question are the background of the researcher, how many patients formed the study group, for how many years the 'cure' has been tested and tried, and who financed the study. It is also good to know if the study was undertaken at a recognised centre of excellence and whether it was a randomised control study.

Likewise, be wary of scare stories about medicines — these are sometimes the result of a 'slow news day' or of a rival drug company paying to have an advertisement, in the guise of an article, inserted in the press. Do not stop taking your medicine on such evidence without first discussing this with your physician. The risks stated may not apply to you, or may not exist at all.

Physiotherapy and related physical treatments

Physiotherapy is the use of physical agents and methods — including massage, exercises, manipulation, hydrotherapy and energy (ultrasound, electricity) — to help the body recover from illness or injury. In general, physiotherapy is helpful for musculoskeletal pain rather than for pain coming from the organs of the body, but any pain can cause reflex muscle spasm and you can get very run down and lose your physical strength from illness and pain.

Stretching and strengthening

Just to take some of the mystery out of physiotherapy, here is a simple guide to some of the principles it uses.

Pain or injury causes muscle spasm; the affected muscles tend to get short and stiff. Some joints and ligaments can get stiff too. Eventually there are parts of the body that just don't move freely anymore. At the same time, other parts of the body have to compensate and this may involve having to move too much. They become strained and weakened, and often painful. Some groups of muscles become overstretched and weak.

Where this happens, especially in the spine, everything gets out of balance, which leads to other problems. Imagine if the wheels on your car are out of alignment: the tyres start to wear on one side, there are strains on the axle, the car begins to rattle, the steering is unreliable and, if you respond by avoiding the problems and not driving it, the engine might seize up and rust. If something like this happens to your body you too may end up weakened, immobile and debilitated.

The physiotherapist aims to prevent or reverse this by stretching tight muscles, freeing up tight joints and ligaments, strengthening weak muscles, and getting you as fit as you can be. At first she does the stretches and movements for you, but later you can do them yourself. One of the most important things about attending physiotherapy sessions is to learn how to become independent and how to stretch and strengthen these muscle groups yourself, creating a 'girdle' of support around the injured or weakened area.

Energy therapies

Even though these are not the sole preserve of the physiotherapist, you are most likely to encounter them in a physiotherapist's rooms. A range of these treatments has been used over the years; the list includes infrared, ultrasound, pulsed short wave, Faradism, Galvanism, and inferential therapy.

There has been speculation about how — and whether — these treatments work to reduce pain especially from soft-tissue injuries. It is likely that they do one or all of the following: increase blood flow to the area (possibly flushing out the inflammatory chemicals that cause pain); reduce painful muscle spasm, and damp down the transmission of pain signals in the spinal cord by 'gating' (see page 13).

Gating is thought to be the way TENS (transcutaneous electrical nerve stimulation, transcutaneous meaning 'across the skin') functions. These machines often bring relief, but do not always work. You can get TENS for use at home. Many pharmacies hire the machines for a trial period, or you can buy one at moderate cost.

'Heat' treatment at home

People sometimes forget you can help relieve pain cheaply at home doing some simple things that may be just as effective as TENS. Over-the-counter ointments like Dencorub and Tiger Balm probably help with pain by increasing blood flow, reducing muscle spasm and by 'gating'. Muscle spasm can be helped by a hot shower or a long hot bath. Bath salts are good if you like them — and just liking them is probably enough to help you relax. Tension is poison.

Just a warning: long hot baths and showers do dry out the skin, which can get itchy and keep you awake at night, or even cause dermatitis (red, itchy, inflamed skin). This can happen to anyone who takes long hot baths and showers especially in winter, which is why it is called 'winter eczema'. If you need to take baths and showers for your pain, avoid using soap on your skin; instead use something like Sorbolene to wash and moisturise your skin. It is an inexpensive and perfectly effective product.

The hot water bottle or heat pack is an important standby, and especially in winter you should keep well rugged up, particularly around the neck because cold causes muscles to tighten up which causes shivering. This is particularly important during the night, and you may find it helps to keep the room slightly warmer than when you are not in pain or experiencing muscle spasms.

5

Caring for Your Mind

Loneliness is one of the unseen pains of illness. This usually arises due to the fact that you cannot leave the house as frequently as you did before and therefore you do not even meet with casual acquaintances in shops nor see friends and neighbours who are out at work full-time. Sitting at home contemplating your situation is probably one of the worst ways of treating pain. If you are no longer able to work but are able to leave the house occasionally, it is a good idea to involve yourself in one of the many volunteer organisations that will be only too happy to welcome you.

Another common reason for aloneness is when people get depressed. Among the features of depression are: losing interest in other activities, avoiding company, being unable to cope with ordinary routines of life and finding no joy from otherwise pleasurable activities. In this situation, it may be very difficult to face getting out of the house. Yet doctors, close friends, dear family and especially the pain sufferer may fail to recognise depression, and it is important to keep an eye out for its warning signs (see page 68).

What must be taken into account is that if you are suffering from pain over a long period of time you may suffer from related depression. This may be due partly to an inability to do what you used to do, but also a sense of catastrophe, in which you make things seem worse than they really are, from fear and avoidance. Unless you find an outlet for your energies and mental challenges and learn to shift the focus away from yourself, you can become unnecessarily preoccupied with your own problems, which may cause you to be hyper-vigilant and reluctant to enter into social activities for fear of 'being different' from the person you once were. The answer lies, to a good degree, in the way you choose to handle the condition.

Psychiatric and psychological treatments

Your experience of pain is influenced by your emotions, expectations and fears and the ways you think about pain. The manner in which you organise your life is a powerful way of responding to pain. Chronic pain can cause problems such as anxiety and depression, which are not only distressing in themselves but also make it harder to cope with very real pain.

Do not fall into the trap of feeling insulted if someone suggests you see a psychologist or psychiatrist. It doesn't mean they think your pain is in your head or that you are a malingerer. It is helpful to have an idea how psychiatric and psychological treatments can help people suffering pain. Remember pain *is* in your head, inasmuch as it is experienced within the brain itself by its clever processing methods.

Depression and anxiety

Especially if anxiety and depression take a hold, a caring and thorough doctor may seek the advice of a psychiatrist who can help decide if medications may be appropriate to help you cope with these problems. Everyone feels low and sad at times, and this is a part of normal life. However, if feeling depressed in response to unfortunate events and situations persists for a long time and pervades every aspect of your life, this can be paralysing and self-perpetuating. With the best will and all the courage in the world, it may be impossible to pull out of this vicious cycle without help from a professional.

It is as if the wagon wheels of your thoughts and feelings keep running in deep ruts, digging them deeper and preventing you from steering the wagon anywhere else. This is rightly referred to as 'major depression', and is probably associated with changes in the chemicals of the nerve cells of the brain. This is where antidepressants can help, by pulling your thoughts and feeling out of those ruts and giving them, and the chemicals of the brain, a chance to become more normal again.

A typical course of antidepressants lasts six months or more.

A psychiatrist may also prescribe antidepressants for anxiety. At first this may seem surprising, since you would think anxiety is almost the opposite of being depressed, and indeed the sorts of doses of antidepressants that are good for depression can make anxiety worse. However, anxiety and depression are flipsides of the same coin. Lower doses of antidepressants are often helpful for anxiety and may be preferable to using the diazepam-based medicines described earlier, which may lead to you requiring increased doses to obtain the same relief from your anxiety.

Psychotherapy

Sometimes deep-seated psychological problems that may be related to events in your past make it harder to cope with your current circumstances. One example of this is post-traumatic stress disorder, which can happen after people have had a terrifying experience. They suffer flashbacks, reliving the experience, and need to avoid anything that might set off the trauma all over again. Post-traumatic stress disorder is often suffered by those who have been involved in an accident or a war, and by rape and assault victims.

Luckily I didn't develop such a problem after my own near-death experience. Maybe it was due to the fact that I had a young baby to live for and was therefore able to change my focus totally. Personally, I have preferred to put my own traumatic disturbances behind me, rather than discussing them with psychologists and psychiatrists. I feel fortunate that it does not appear to have been necessary for me. But for some people, psychotherapy may be the preferred or necessary method. A qualified psychiatrist or psychologist is the only professional to see. Check that psychiatrists and psychologists are members of an appropriate professional college and have the appropriate registration.

Bear in mind that not all psychiatrists are interested in doing psychotherapy. It is time-consuming, and they may practice as physicians using psychoactive medicines rather than as counsellors. You may need to look around to find a psychiatrist who is trained in and committed to this kind of work, especially if you can't afford to pay a private psychologist.

Hopefully your GP will be able to help you find the right person if you need supportive counselling or psychotherapy, because it can be very distressing to tell your life story to someone then to find he is only interested in giving you pills. People get very dispirited having to go from one therapist to another to discover what they need, and their range of choices may be limited by the cost of private treatment.

Remember that no clairvoyant or faith healer, however well meaning, is able to prescribe medication, or assess the entire clinical picture. And many people call themselves counsellors without having certified qualifications.

Cognitive behavioural therapy (CBT)

Cognitive behavioural therapy (CBT) is offered by qualified psychologists. It sounds complicated, but the principles behind it are not so difficult to grasp. A person in pain may have *thoughts* on the lines of 'There's no point me going out, I'll only be in pain and I won't enjoy myself, and everyone will avoid me anyway.' They may also get into the habit of behaving in some ways that are unhelpful, such as limping in a certain way or spending the day in bed, to avoid pain.

This therapy is not about blaming you for your own pain: after all, it might be perfectly reasonable to think there is no point in going out, and quite understandable to limp. The aim of CBT is to help identify ways of thinking and behaving that are self-perpetuating and counter-productive, challenge them, and consciously and deliberately change them so that you can cope.

CBT can help people with chronic pain. These are techniques that have also been shown to be effective for some types of anxiety and for helping people stay off drugs. CBT helps you harness your strengths and is one of the few psychological treatments that has survived the test of randomised trials. It teaches you such simple things as getting out and about, which may ultimately help you to cope better, and trying to avoid limping, which may spare your hips and spine as well as making you feel more positive about yourself. Walk tall and proudly if you can — it does much for your self-image.

You learn ways of thinking and behaving and tend to stick with them. It's not so easy to unlearn things. For some it might be as simple as 'thinking positively' and 'looking on the bright side', but very often it is a great deal more complex than that. Having a professional to work through these things really helps.

A note about alcohol

May I stress that alcohol and medicines do not mix. Particularly if you are taking prescribed opioids or antihistamines, you may suffer severe side effects far worse than the pain you may be attempting to block. Personally, one-third of a glass of champagne makes my head feel as if it is going to explode. Most medicines carry warnings against combination with alcohol, but like all warnings to which you become accustomed it is easy not to pay any attention to them.

6

Complementary and Alternative Therapies

Before you consult any new therapist, it is a good idea to check the official government registration board (if there is one) to ensure your choice is of a practitioner who is fully qualified and recognised. This is not just to protect your health; it may also save you financially. It is important and comforting to note that in order to advertise professional services in a telephone directory, one must comply with the regulations stating essential registration to an approved and recognised professional body.

An increasing number of health funds are including 'complementary' medical techniques. Among those considered for refund are: acupuncture, reflexology, chiropractic and osteopathy. Some of these have been regarded as mainstream for years, as are homeopathy, hypnotherapy and some of the 'softer' new age therapies such as aromatherapy and massage. (Interestingly, in France, complementary alternative medicine is referred to as *la médecine douce* or sweet/soft medicine.)

As a starting point, you might be guided by personal recommendations from a trusted friend. Consider therapies that involve your body and mind: meditation, creative visualisation, yoga, music therapy, aquarobics, Pilates, Feldenkrais and the Alexander technique.

Several of these alternative or complementary approaches may be helpful in managing pain. This is not an attempt to be definitive or exhaustive but is intended to orient you a little before you make your own enquiries. Because alternative therapies are so many and varied, I will not attempt to explain their benefits or advantages. There is a suggested reading list at the end of the book (see page 219).

Selected alternative therapies

Acupuncture

This is one of the treatments that straddles alternative and western medicine, partly because it has been *the* mainstream medicine in such a large part of the world for such a long time, and also because it has found its way into western medicine as well, albeit within limits.

Nowadays most doctors would agree that acupuncture can help with treating pain. Film footage of complex operations being carried out without anaesthetics and with the patient's pain and discomfort being managed by acupuncture alone is very impressive and enough to dumbfound any sceptic. Gating theory provides a theoretical basis for acupuncture reducing pain.

The techniques of acupuncture were developed empirically (that is, by observation, trial and error) over millennia, and their concept of 'meridians' (regions of the body) and 'flows of energy' ties it all up into a neat model. This is where western medicine may beg to differ: you can accept that acupuncture is doing something effective without necessarily believing there is any such thing as a meridian, at least in the human body.

Just because the ancients could pinpoint the movements of planets and stars, it doesn't mean that Aristotle's model of circles and spheres were more than symbols for the real process that was going on. Not until Newton and others cottoned on to the idea of gravity did we humans begin to understand how and why it was all happening.

When a respected surgeon at a pain clinic first suggested to me that I receive acupuncture as regular treatment for pain relief following cervical (neck) surgery, I was reassured that he believed that acupuncture would be suitable for keeping pain at bay post-surgically. However, I was fearful and more ready to accept the services of a GP who also practised acupuncture. I found a local doctor who could offer me this. After a couple of sessions, dignified and honourable as he was, he admitted having only undergone a very short course of study and that my condition was too complex to benefit from his treatment. It was outside his realm of experience or preparation. Of itself, this was interesting and I was grateful for his honesty. In fact, his application of nine needles to certain points gave me little relief from severe pain. He also treated me for only twenty minutes per session.

A trusted friend recommended a marvellous acupuncturist who had given her great relief over years of severe pain. He was qualified in acupuncture only, had forty-two years experience and had trained in Japan, where he had worked for ten years prior to coming to Australia. I was amazed when he inserted approximately a hundred needles each session, which lasted ninety minutes and cost less than a long GP consultation (it may be partly recompensed by some health funds). The ensuing short-term relief, the reassurance and occasional total relief from pain was phenomenal.

Western medicine wins every time as far as understanding physical processes in the body and has developed some very powerful treatments as a result. Nevertheless, a conventional doctor may be very puzzled about how an acupuncture needle in the hand can make the foot twitch on the opposite side of the body, all the more so if she experiences it herself. The process going on is obviously a lot more complex than gating — which is not really surprising, given the complexities of the nervous system.

Beyond providing analgesia by gating pain, it may be that acupuncture can also relieve muscle spasm and release some of those shortened muscles that set the musculoskeletal system out of alignment. By helping to restore balance in the function of certain nerves, muscles and joints, it could be doing rather more than just temporarily blocking pain. If you have ever felt your sinuses suddenly empty with the insertion of the ninth acupuncture needle, you might wonder if they might just be able to clear out your gallbladder in the same way.

This is a gentler and more holistic way of restoring balance to the body than manipulating the spine. And it is safe and free of side effects, provided the therapist is using disposable needles.

If for most organic diseases it could be wisest to choose

western medicine, the term 'complementary therapy' seems to fit acupuncture well.

Chiropractic and osteopathy

It is difficult to separate these two without going into extensive detail. Simple definitions won't do it as there are different schools of both chiropractic and osteopathy, and some practitioners are qualified in both.

The difference is in the physical techniques used. Like physiotherapists, osteopaths and chiropractors should spend a substantial amount of time stretching shortened muscles and ligaments and working substantially with manual massage and other 'soft-tissue' treatments before performing any manipulations of the body joint. They tend to do fewer if any physical exercises to strengthen muscles and concentrate more on manipulation.

Most of the evidence of benefit from these techniques is anecdotal, although some proper studies have been done, and the evidence is getting better: for example, results from an excellent Dutch study showing the benefit of 'neck mobilisation' were recently published in the *British Medical Journal*. It makes sense that chiropractic and osteopathic techniques should help with certain types of musculoskeletal pain. As these practitioners concentrate on the idea of functional disturbance rather than on disease, they may have an advantage over doctors, who are sometimes at a bit of a loss when there is no actual *pathology*.

A medical dictionary defines osteopathy as 'a system of therapy using normal medical principles of diagnosis but aiming to allow the body to treat itself by restoring good structural balance, healthy environment and nutrition'. The emphasis is on good body mechanics and correcting structural imbalances by such methods as manipulation. The idea is that if the 'chassis' of the body is out of ideal balance, blood and lymph won't flow freely, nerve impulses will be distorted, and so on.

As with physiotherapy, there are exercises and stretches you should do at home. Ask for advice and printed handouts on this. It is easy to be a bit lazy and happy to let others work on your body, but if these techniques are to work you should follow up with suitable exercises at home. It may save money, too.

Chiropractic deals with the diagnosis, treatment and prevention of mechanical disorders of the musculoskeletal system, and the effects of these disorders on the functions of the nervous system and general health. There is an emphasis on manual treatments, including spinal adjustment and other joint and soft-tissue manipulation. People consult a chiropractor for spinal symptoms (neck and back pain), headaches, migraines and sciatica, and for relief from asthma, sinusitis and digestive disorders.

As with all health practitioners, chiropractors vary in their practice styles and focus. Some have further qualifications or interests in specific areas, such as paediatrics, sports injuries or rehabilitation. Some practitioners use 'manipulative' techniques, others use Activator or kinesiology-based methods. Chiropractors should also be able to coach you in lifestyle changes, including ergonomic advice, exercises, stretches, and so on.

Do not be afraid to ask questions of a practitioner before you choose who to go to. Like dentists and GPs, some are more suitable for certain people than others. You do not need a referral from a doctor and in most cases you can claim costs if treatment is related to a compensable injury.

Massage

Of course massage helps relieve some sorts of pain, for all the reasons already explored. Massage may relieve pain through gating but probably most benefits come from stretching out shortened muscle fibres and ligaments. And for people who live alone and who are seldom touched, the mere touching by another caring person can have a comforting placebo effect. But massage is not going to cure cancer.

Be aware that the most painful massage isn't necessarily the most effective one, despite the masochistic pleasure it may give you. If it makes you 'guard' against the pain by increasing muscle tension, it may make things worse.

Pilates

Pilates, named after its founder, is an exercise system to develop the strength and balance of the muscles that support the body: the muscles holding up the spine and pelvis. Most of us probably don't even know they are there. Theoretically, Pilates would be expected to have some benefits for people with various types of musculoskeletal pains, and as a way of building general strength and resilience.

An interesting aspect of the method is that Pilates developed a lot of elaborate machines to help train all those muscles to tip-top perfection. Whether that was out of a fascination with technology and the body perfect — it was the 1920s and 1930s

— or a desire to establish a brand image for his technique (he migrated to America where he made his fortune), one might wonder whether all that ironmongery is really necessary.

Alexander technique

Named after its founder, this postural technique aims to achieve functional and structural balance by retraining you in more natural ways of using the body. F M Alexander blamed humans' upright posture for many of our ills: gravity tends to make us distort the use of our bodies, unlike fish and four-legged animals, who move sleekly and smoothly, he argued. So it is not just about posture, but how we move. At the time Alexander (who was Tasmanian) became all the rage in smart circles in London in the 1930s there was much fascination with Charles Sherrington's research on the nervous system. Sherrington's experiments with cats proved that the muscles and orientation of the neck are important in the balance and coordination of the body.

In theory, the Alexander technique is one of the most holistic ways of dealing with musculoskeletal ills as there is no outside intervention: you just gradually restore balance to your body. Gradually is the operative word — there are no short cuts. The Alexanders call short cuts 'end-gaining'. Actors and singers seem to find the technique beneficial, maybe because they need their necks to be well positioned to optimise the voice box. But, like anything else, there can be too much of a good thing: the term 'Alexandroid' refers to the person who has achieved a very stilted way of moving in a quixotic quest for perfect posture. As for the benefits for chronic pain sufferers, it remains a question mark.

Feldenkrais

The Feldenkrais method is another postural technique designed to improve posture, flexibility, coordination, self-image and to alleviate muscular tension and pain. It uses two approaches: gentle movement to retrain every joint and muscle group in the body and one-on-one manipulation and passive movement sessions. It is advisable to seek a qualified practitioner through those listed in professional directories of specialists who are registered with an appopriate association.

Aquatherapy

Aquatherapy, or hydrotherapy, is now part of mainstream post-surgical healing: it is a standard form of physiotherapy offered by most hospitals, usually at their own facilities. Importantly, the water temperature must be around 34 degrees Centigrade. The water found in public pools will be about 26 degrees Centigrade maximum: this is too cold for muscles which may go into spasm, particularly after the trauma of accident or surgery. Aquatherapy, which is not to be confused with supervised exercises with a physiotherapist, helps patients to strengthen their muscles, which may otherwise become withered if immobilised for even a couple of weeks post-trauma. It has a pleasant relaxing effect which, unfortunately, can lead you to be overactive in the water: it isn't until after you get out of the lovely warm womb-like environment that pain hits in. This can be the experience of many people keen to get strong again too rapidly.

But used wisely it is valuable. It was thrilling for me to see a woman in her fifties who four weeks earlier had undergone spinal surgery — fusion of L4+5, L 2+3 (L stands for lumbar, T for tho-racic and C for cervical when referring to the vertebrae) — walking in the comfortably heated swimming pool (35°C) at our local hospital facility. To my amazement she walked out of the water, dressed herself, and then walked up the hill to the bus carrying a backpack. In contrast, when I had similar surgery eighteen years before, I was kept flat on my back for six weeks. When I left hospital I had to wear a metal brace, was not permitted to drive, could not walk more than fifty metres without crutches and suffered considerable pain for several months. This woman told me she was practically pain-free. This encouraging story goes to show how far advances in medicine and medical practice have come in a relatively short time.

Herbal remedies

Herbal remedies do not undergo the same scrutiny as prescription medicines. The way they may interact with your doctor's carefully measured drug dosages may cause the prescription medicine to be less effective or may bring on a sensitivity that may actually harm you. St John's Wort is an example of a 'natural' substance that can adversely affect other medicines. Some people choose herbal rem-edies simply because they like the notion of the word 'herbal', and they drink herbal teas because they sound 'virtuous' and 'healthy'. There is nothing wrong with a chamomile tea with honey at night-time to ease you into a gentle sleep. Whether it is likely to induce sleep or not is 'all in the mind'. Of course, that is what really matters.

Just because herbs are 'natural' does not mean they can be

used indiscriminately and nor does it mean they are harm-free. Herbs have been used to brew powerful, even lethal, poisons throughout history — careful study of everything you take is essential. Most pharmacists can give you valuable advice on the wisdom and dangers of combining substances, so seek advice and never take something simply because a friend says it works. Our bodies are all so biochemically different, and there is no reason Bill's sleeping herbs will be good for you or that Jane's herbal cough remedy will or won't be suitable if you suffer from asthma or take other prescription medications.

Spirituality

This book is for everyone, regardless of religious affiliations or belief systems. Your belief system is built on many different levels, some from childhood, or experience, disbelief, or some magnificent vision that has inspired and given you strength and courage. Often a person can lead you in that direction, or a book, a mentor or an event can.

You may choose to be guided by the spiritual strength of mind and body, the study of philosophy and the wisdom of great thinkers such as Descartes, Pascal, Gandhi, Bernie Siegel and Deepak Chopra. Their philosophy (which should be available in different forms of media) may assist you in coming to terms with aspects of illness you are unable to comprehend. If you can briefly leave your body through meditation and concentration, you can often dull some of the more rigorous sessions of pain instead of using less positive ways, such as smoking or over-indulgence in alcohol.

Meditation

Again, with the idea that your mental and emotional state can affect your experience of pain, meditation is sure to benefit some people. There are plenty of cultural examples of people gaining strength from meditation, and many types of meditation to choose.

One word of caution though. If you are bed-ridden and fatigued as a result of your pain, too much meditation can sometimes make you too inwardly focused. So meditation may be better for pain as such, than for chronic fatigue.

Yoga

Yoga is a lot more than a 'treatment'. It has both mental and spiritual elements that may alter your perception of pain. It also promotes balanced function of the body and increases flexibility and strength. There is every reason in the world to expect that this would be beneficial if you have chronic or recurrent pain. It may also be a good way of getting out of the house and meeting people. Once again, choose your yoga teacher through an appropriate professional, registered organisation.

Music therapy

Music therapy can play an important part in helping children to release their thoughts and express themselves. Those who study methods of assisting children in this way believe that through participation and by joining in the children's world of pain or suffering, they can lead them towards a happier and more accepting understanding of all that is happening to them, relieving any 'guilt for being sick' — a notion from which many children suffer intolerable additional unhappiness.

Music therapy as a passive, listening exercise can be useful, of course, but what is even more effective for a child, who may dread the length of each day in hospital, is to become fully involved in an activity such as songwriting, in which he can use words to express anger, pain, desolation, guilt and abandonment under the guidance of a specialist therapist. Listening can form part of his meditative plan, as can resting or simply lying still, when the mind can form its own pictures according to the audio stimulation from a symphony, a pop song, some tune or jingle.

You can watch small children under three lying in their cots humming or tapping away merrily in their own little world of music. The Suzuki method of teaching very young babies and children through participation and involving the parents will help in their rehabilitation. Suzuki teachers should be accredited.

Music therapy can also play an important part in an adult's experience, both in hospital and at home. Various styles of music are used — not necessarily by trained therapists, sometimes by those who love music and have something to offer — and many patients, particularly those whose speech is impaired by illness, respond positively to this. You may even choose to take up the study of an instrument and discover the therapeutic value of this skill, which will also help to distract you from your pain, provided you do not overdo things and develop RSI by over-keen practice.

Art therapy

Parents tend to be overjoyed as soon as a child is given paper and crayons and can construct an image. Initially, it is absurd to read too much into these images of mum, dad, the house or the family pet. But, particularly with children who cannot or will not express themselves verbally, an entire construct of what is happening at home can gradually emerge through draw-the-family pictures and various entertaining but telling exercises set by the trained art therapist. The colours chosen will have significance or may simply be used because they are all that are available. A small percentage of children may be colour blind, which can also explain odd choices of colour (boys have a higher incidence of colour blindness than girls, about ten times higher). Drawings can be a useful way of opening a conversation with verbal children. Enjoyment and pleasure may be expressed, as will anger, rage and humour.

The draw-a-man test has long been used by educational psychologists as a measuring device for intelligence. But many question the value of this test for children over ten, as it can be interpreted deviously both by child and practitioner and may signify nothing more than boredom, anger or disinterest.

Over a six-month period I learned more about the autistic children in my care through art combined with music as a background than by any other method. I would play a piece of music they knew, such as 'Yellow Submarine', and then give out the paper and crayons. These children, all aged under twelve with attention spans seldom exceeding five minutes, would construct something from the theme, and quite frequently it was yellow and resembled a boat. The rest of the time was spent in one-to-one work, while the other children would sit away from each other (I taught in groups not exceeding four at a time). All the children were non-verbal. Many screamed when not engaged in specific activities and others self-abused. But art and music calmed them briefly and that was the only time we could work as a group. These sessions were a useful means of communication: the children could show me their anger, rage (violent scribblings and dark colours) or happiness (usually a bright representation of the sun, or of a pretty flower).

Choosing your treatment

Any of these ways of helping your pain may be useful. It is advisable to find out more about the type you are attracted to: why it was started, by whom, how successful the method appears to be and the way that success has been measured (from proper studies or purely on anecdotal evidence). If you can afford to, it may not matter that you simply enjoy experimenting, but if you are very unwell, just tramping from one session to another can be as exhausting as the benefits gained. Bear in mind the possible benefits and limitations of each method, and do some homework. The internet is the most accessible source. Here are some questions to investigate:

- How long has the therapy been used, who evolved the method and why?
- What benefits are claimed for it and by whom?
- How long a training course do the therapists undertake, what qualifications do they earn and is there a requirement for them to be registered?
- Do major health funds recognise the therapy?

- How many sessions do various conditions require before improvement is noted?
- The limitations and risks involved in the therapy.

As mentioned earlier, practitioners of many therapies need to be registered. The official website of the registering board should be your first port of call when choosing a therapist. And seek the advice of your GP or specialist advisor when you need to find new information on services connected with the very important subject of your health.

By searching on the internet you can establish most of the information you need. Most websites will also give you addresses of practitioners, list their registration and give you a map so you know how to get there and where to park. You can phone the practice and ask to speak with the person who will offer the service.

If the therapist is unwilling to explain these things before you have a treatment, perhaps that particular service provider is not for you.

Be aware that some websites contain news items from cranks who wish to see their opinions published but who have little or no true experience or expertise.

Please don't stumble along to every class you see advertised. Your medical specialist may have a particular reason against your joining in over-active exercises and certain movements could further worsen your condition. Just check things out and see what is on offer. Keeping an open mind is vital, particularly if western medicine has not been able to offer you on-going help.

Bernie Siegel, the American physician who has written many valuable books on ways of coping with cancer, considers that any treatment modality his patients choose, providing they choose it with 'positive conviction' and not 'out of fear', is likely to be right for them. But if the patient says, 'I am scared to death of surgery', and therefore chooses something else, Siegel cannot support that choice because, as he stresses in his book *Love, Medicine, and Miracles*, 'Treatment chosen out of that type of fear is unlikely to be successful. A patient must understand that "all healing is scientific".' It is your hope and the changes you produce when you are on the therapy that produces the results. The most important thing is to believe in the therapy and proceed with a positive attitude.

Bear in mind that the choice must be yours. That is the message Siegel gives you. This dedicated oncologist is respected and revered by the many patients who benefit from his treatment philosophy. Siegel says that since so many cancer patients feel they have so little control over their lives, making a choice can, of itself, be a turning point. His many groups (known as ECaP or exceptional cancer patient groups) have proved that discussion with others and sharing ideas for a greater understanding can be very empowering too. His books may comfort you and give you a sense of calm understanding.

Siegel's books include *Love, Medicine and Miracles, Peace, Love and Healing, How to Live Between Office Visits* and *Prescriptions for Living*. Many come with tapes, which are a useful resource for calm meditation and for listening to messages that are affirming and helpful, not just for those suffering from cancer but from all forms of illness, pain and distress.

By all means inform yourself about the therapy you are seeking, but remember the dictum: a little knowledge is a dangerous thing. On the internet you will find well researched articles whose provenance is not in doubt (look for authors and publications with acknowledged credibility, such as universities and medical schools, official registration boards, well-known academic journals. Be careful not to take everything you read as gospel.

Discuss it with your medical advisors before you embrace any suggestions involved with 'healing'. You will probably find your doctor is relatively conservative in recommendations. The reason doctors may be against alternative therapies could be well founded. There may be no evidence-based research on the therapy and the practitioners offering it may have paid to undertake a weekend course, then hung out their shingle. It is not fair to assume that doctors are just bloody-minded about competition from comple-mentary or alternative practitioners. Some doctors may be too tough in cases where it is difficult to prove some treatments are beneficial. But you may be so over-eager to 'get well', you rush into the unknown when what your good doctor is trying to do is to protect you from villains. This is why it is important to check the qualifications and experience of your newly sought-out prac-titioner. It is frightening to look up on the internet where courses and degrees can be bought without any course requirements. This is why you must be sure the practitioner's certificate is recognised by the appropriate professional regulatory boards.

Even when you are satisfied you have chosen the right

therapy, unless you know of the practitioner from personal recommendation, you may have to make a little leap of faith on your first visit — there is a limit to how much you can find out without putting your toe in the water.

When trying out a new therapy, find out what you may expect to pay for treatments and how long a session will last. Is special equipment needed, different clothing, a mat and pillow? Use much the same strategy as you devoted to preparing yourself for asking and listening to your doctor. Give the therapist brief notes explaining your condition, your medical history, allergies or past problems encountered, and weigh up the atmosphere of the practice, the people it attracts, and the interaction of staff members.

So follow these principles when considering alternative therapies:

- get informed and ask for personal recommendation from friends
- discuss the therapy with your GP
- weigh up costs and benefits (include financial costs and risks)
- if unsure, there may be a case for trial and and error.

Once you've begun a course of therapy, try to be as objective as possible about its effectiveness. If at any stage you feel that it is aggrevating your condition and/or increasing your pain, stop immediately.

Magnetic therapy: Renée's story, part II

There has been a recent vogue for wearing magnets embedded in material and in belts around the area in pain (back belts, shoulder braces) as well as magnet-filled mattress overlays. Some people swear by the wearing of bracelets that have magnets within them.

No study has given satisfactory science-based evidence as to whether these devices are effective or not. If you do decide to experiment with magnetism, try a product with a money-back guarantee. There is anecdotal evidence of patients reporting good results — which may be due to some faith in the person who recommended the product or to a 'placebo' response.

There is a definite but rather unusual use for a magnet which my medical advisors recommended when I was living in France. This is a type of embedded TENS machine and was developed initially for use in pain reduction for patients who were suffering from multiple sclerosis.

The implanted TENS has a varied therapeutic history and is recommended by some neurological specialists. Some studies have reported it to be effective for some patients some of the time. Recent research in Britain showed a less than 30 per cent favourable response beyond four years of use. As the device is costly and involves surgical implant, it is not widely used except when almost everything else has failed to alleviate painful symptoms.

The device works by distracting the signals of pain on their way to the brain and confusing them (the gating method). In my case, the operation to install the stimulator was carried out at the University of Toulouse and involved the insertion of electrodes in my spinal canal. To these were attached fine wires that protruded from two sites: one in my front, the other in the back. The front one was the escape hatch for a device the size of a television remote control.

The stimulator was set in motion by means of a large blue magnet about the size of a small mobile phone. There were only two settings, 'on' and 'off' (nowadays there is a more sophisticated version that controls the strength of the signals). To make the machine work, the magnet was passed across the electronic pain-relieving stimulator embedded under the ribcage. When I felt a sensation that was like hundreds of crawling ants constantly creeping up and down my legs, I knew that the machine was on and that my brain was to be tricked into deferring — distracting — pain messages.

On one occasion I lost my magnet and was overwhelmed with panic because the machine was off and, as I was experiencing considerable pain, I dearly needed it to be on. A friend lent me her kindergarten child's large black and white cow magnet. I was delighted that it worked. The magnet amused those who saw me dragging it out of my handbag, so I bought myself an even funnier one, a bright pink Miss Piggy. But the trouble with that — and indeed with any other magnet — was its ability to erase the magnetic strip from my credit cards as well as causing other havoc, in all kinds of circumstances.

In due course, the stimulator failed to control pain and the only solution was to remove it. My consultant admitted that it was unclear exactly how the pain stimulator did achieve pain relief or why it had failed.

My machine did afford me blessed relief from my back pain,

which the twelve previous surgical interventions had not managed to quell, for two out of the four years it was embedded. More recent devices are smaller, the internal segment being no larger than a large coat button and the on-off control is about the size of a tiny mobile telephone and can be carried discreetly in a little belt or phone pouch. Alas, as my body rejected the implant, neurologists seem to agree that implanting another would be likely to fail also. Everything is not suitable for everyone.

During my years in France, my experience with a magnet caused much embarrassment, particularly with cutlery. One evening we were dining at an elegant establishment in Paris, but when I rose to leave the table, my big black leather handbag in which the magnet was hidden managed to attach itself to a sterling silver fork. A somewhat bewildered maître d'hôtel summoned his security guard and it was with considerable difficulty that I explained how I apparently had come to 'lift' one of the valuable silver pieces from the table.

The only article I totally destroyed was an audio cassette. Naturally, the cassette was the story of a thriller, which I hadn't finished listening to so I shall never know whodunit.

7

Lifting Your Spirits

This chapter is all about ways of using your own strengths in the management of your pain. One of the best ways of raising your self-esteem is to understand that you do have a part to play in your own pain control. This empowers you and gives you confidence. Often, by helping others, you will simply forget your own problems, albeit briefly.

Distraction

A very important way of combating pain is distraction, a method well documented by research. In contrast, focusing on pain may intensify it.

Nerve fibres throughout the body are constantly monitoring for pain. Pain is a helpful signal for the body: for example, when it warns you to get away from a hot object, to change your posture at the computer so you do not get neck or shoulder pain, or even during sleep to cause you to roll over so you do not develop a bed sore. Most of the time these constant messages from pain fibres are subconscious and you don't notice them. Try this experiment: if you are sitting, let yourself become aware of the mild pain coming from where your bottom is in contact with the chair. Similarly, you might like to notice the itch sensation which is probably coming from your socks or underclothes without you being aware of it — usually you pay no attention to these constant subtle 'itch' signals from parts of your body. (But don't concentrate on your natural itch sensations too much, or they might begin to drive you crazy.)

Some important physiological studies have shown that pain sensations can be reduced or blocked by a different nerve stimulus feeding in at around the same level of the spinal cord where the pain is located: gating theory forms the basis of many medical treatments for pain using nerve stimulation.

It is also very easy to become self-obsessed when you suffer from chronic pain. If you keep occupied and are happy with what you do, you will have less time or inclination to concentrate on your pain and discomfort. But you must learn the importance of pacing your activities so you do not become over-tired, which is counter-productive.

Your fear of isolation from the mainstream will alter as you become more productive. If you have been a very active person and your illness has slowed you down, you will have suffered from the change in your daily routine. One of the things you might like to do is to create a timetable for yourself with aims and objectives for each day. It's best to keep these lists modest, because you do not want to have to deal with a sense of failure by not meeting your own self-imposed objectives. If each day you can achieve even one thing on your list, you will gain satisfaction from that alone.

Your self-esteem may also have taken a battering from your inability to do the things you used to, and you may even find yourself questioning whether or not you are really ill. If you have one of the many illnesses that are without exterior signs, such as backache or multiple sclerosis (in its early stages), unkind people may even suggest that you are not really ill and are pretending in order to avoid work or gain attention. But who would choose the life of an invalid over that of being an active member of society?

You have to learn to become resilient against those who doubt you and, rather than defend yourself, demonstrate by your own efforts that you do your best. You soon discover your true friends: when you are sick and in pain, you do not have time to deal with acquaintances or people who are judgemental and critical all the time.

For children, the absence of companions can be devastating, and it is difficult for parents to be there constantly to ensure fair play or amusement. Parents of children with psychiatric illnesses will be familiar with the loss of many a previous 'friend' who announces definitively that 'your children only behave that way because you brought them up badly'. Such comments are not only hurtful and unfair but make life even harder for the unfortunate parent whose coping mechanisms are daily challenged with family life already. You need your friends through thick and thin — and you must cast away those who are fair-weather friends.

Humour and laughter

Laughter is good for all of us. Thomas Merton, the great Trappist monk, was famous for his sense of humour. He put into words his feelings about the seriousness of religion, saying how great it was to be contemplating the beauties of nature, and by looking at the sky realising how small everything else is, including 'all the solemn stuff' spoken 'by professional asses' in the name of philosophy or religion. You can, of course, take yourself far too seriously.

The ability to laugh at your own helplessness in pain produces some great endorphins which aid with pain reduction. That 'hearty' laugh is also good for your heart as it stimulates the circulation. In the book *Laughter Therapy,* Annette Goodheart explains how the simple act of laughing releases important chemicals that ease pain.

A word of caution. You can actually be cruel when you don't mean to be by taking things a little too far: one example is of tickling, which can be distressing — it *can* lead to good laughter that is healing but it can also lead to pain, clenched muscles and embarrassment.

Smile more

Like laughing, the physical act of smiling releases endorphins into our brains. The endorphins are nature's opiates, they make you feel good and can be likened to pleasure-producing chemicals.

One American psychologist believed it possible to cure depression simply by teaching patients to smile more. His theory has been investigated and reported in papers published in medical journals. What these researchers found is that smiling is good for you physiologically as well as emotionally. Try smiling next time you are feeling low. The scientific reason it makes you feel better is that the movement of facial muscles involved causes a pattern of constriction and the release of facial blood vessels. This changes the flow of blood to the brain, fractionally altering its temperature, which then triggers the release of endorphins and suppresses the release of other brain chemicals. According to a French study, smiling strengthens the immune system.

Smiling uses thirteen facial muscles, whereas frowning uses more than forty muscles, so smiling is an excellent anti-ageing device, as the facial skin of smilers is usually smoother than that of frowners. Quite a useful beauty tip.

A smile costs nothing, but gives much. It enriches those
who receive, without making poorer those who give.
It takes but a moment, but the memory of it sometimes
lasts forever. None is so rich or mighty that he can get
along without it, and none is so poor that he can't be made
rich by it. A smile creates happiness in the home, fosters
goodwill in business and is the countersign of friendship.
It brings rest to the weary, cheer to the discouraged,
sunshine to the sad and it is nature's best antidote for
troubles. Yet it cannot be bought, begged, borrowed or
stolen, for it is something that is of no value to anyone
until it is given away. Some people are too tired to give
you a smile. Give them one of yours, as none need to smile
so much as he who has no more to give.

— *Anon*

The point is, you can choose to smile, you can practise it. Wheelchair patients are forced to smile to get anything done, and also to prove to those around them that they are not 'idiots' and are worth speaking to.

Do not concern yourself about those who accuse you of smiling falsely — that is pedantic. It means at least that you are attempting to show goodwill to those to whom you offer that smile. Only with your loved ones can you afford to admit defeat — except, of course, in therapeutic medical situations. The saying 'Smile and the world smiles with you, cry and you cry alone' is still pretty true today.

Eating well

When you are sick or in pain, one of the things that can easily be overlooked is nutrition. Often appetite is lacking, particularly in the presence of nausea — a common side effect of medication — and it can be difficult to eat anything at all.

People suffering from constipation need particular advice. Constipation is one of the side effects of opioids and of itself can cause significant head pain, a feeling of bloating, stomach pains, cramps and fullness. Various products can ease this, among them over-the-counter remedies from your pharmacist, including Movicol, fruit-based 'natural' laxatives, fibre-rich products that help to fill and push the material through the gut, and Coloxyl which will soften the faeces and assist pushing when muscles may be weak from surgical procedures or scar tissue. But consult your doctor first, and if the source of your pain is a direct result of an abdominal complication, do not take laxatives without your doctor's knowledge and advice. (Your regular pharmacist should also be aware of the medications you use. If you are on medication for rheumatoid arthritis or osteoporosis, for example, he would know certain calcium-containing supplements are not for you as their interaction with other medicines could prevent you from absorbing the medicine.)

Opioids slow the movement of food through your intestines and this can lead to weight loss in some people. Others put on weight, but this is often due to inactivity and the disability caused by the pain. If your faeces are hard and cause tiny blood vessels to break when you go to the toilet, it's useful to put a handful of Sorbolene cream on your soft toilet tissue (three-ply is recommended) to soften the skin around your bottom, which reduces the tendency to forcing and light bleeding. Severe bleeding is reason enough to visit your doctor, particularly if it happens more than once.

Constipation causes chronic pain if it goes untreated, and so many patients forget to mention it or embarrassment overcomes them when they see their doctor. Some health services fund nurses to assess patients who suffer from chronic pain and live at home. These nurses are experts on constipation, urinary problems and incontinence. Your local GP or community health centre will provide you with the details and possibly arrange the home visit for you. Remember also the healing properties of manuka honey, which is renowned not only for its digestive aids and antibacterial benefits but also for its natural antibiotic properties.

If swallowing is a problem, and there is no one to help you

prepare meals, you may find a protein drink helpful as a substitute meal once a day if the alternative is to forego eating altogether. Products such as Sustagen and Resource Plus, which are readily available, contain protein, vitamins and minerals; be aware, however, that these are not a complete meal substitute. If you do not tolerate milk products, ask your doctor to suggest an alternative protein source.

Try to include five vegetables and three fruits a day, but if you can't prepare these, you can buy vegetables juices and fruit you enjoy. Sometimes the energy needed when you are sick is just too great to expend on cooking. If you are finding it hard to organise meals, you might ask your friends to help prepare them occasionally. When caring for a sick child, you need to go that extra mile to make meals enticing. Small helpings often are best, with little tempting treats such as a boiled egg and 'soldiers' with a thin covering of butter and Marmite, yoghurt and fruit, scrambled eggs, a homemade soup (or quality preparations with organic vegetables and no chemical additives would be acceptable).

For a chronically ill child, it is good to consult a dietician on suitable food containing adequate proteins, vitamins and minerals for the child's age and size, and it is important to ensure your child is well hydrated — a dry tongue is a simple warning sign of under-hydration. A mixture of fluids is best: some of it water, some fresh fruit juice, some drinks with electrolytes (such as soda water, mineral water or other carbonated drinks).

There is never a substitute for fresh vegetables and fruit, and perhaps a sick child will be happy if you mash or blend these in a palatable, easy-to-swallow drink to maximise fresh vitamins.

Time-consuming though it may be, try to prepare these drinks frequently, perhaps in batches which last for twenty-four hours — after that they lose peak nutrition. If your child is dehydrated or vomiting, you will of course seek the advice of your doctor. It may be necessary for the child to be hospitalised and fed intravenously to re-hydrate as efficiently as possible, albeit briefly. Tiny bodies dehydrate rapidly. Usually oral rehydration is adequate and there are quite good products available that provide the necessary minerals and energy. Unfortunately, severe pain can, of itself, cause nausea, vomiting and, as a result, dehydration.

When you are ill, you should attend to your body's additional needs for vitamins and mineral supplements. If you can build up the immune system, you will fight infection better and also cope with pain more effectively. The body works hard with all its mechanisms when you are in pain, so you need extra help, particularly at such times. A multi-vitamin pill designed for a specific age group or condition is readily available and can be a good adjunct, but taking unnecessary supplements can cause unpleasant side effects and be a waste of money. Ask your chemist for advice.

Many of the great foods are the simplest ones. Porridge oats are easily and quickly cooked on top of the stove or in the microwave and with a piece of fruit make a wholesome breakfast. Or eat muesli. Heal your body with whole foods whenever possible, using pineapples, mangos and bananas as well as good fresh green vegetables. Choose those that are organically produced if possible because ingesting pesticides and other chemicals is the last thing you need. If your child is able to eat raw vegetables such as grated carrots, these are much more valuable nutritionally than when cooked, but they might be difficult to digest for children who are unable to chew them well.

When eating is aggravating pain or causing discomfort, naturally you lose your appetite. Soon not eating at all becomes the norm. It is important to recognise the signs of anorexia nervosa, a severe eating disorder usually suffered by young people perceiving themselves to be excessively fat even if they are underweight. When nausea as a result of pain causes a dislike of all food, be wary of patients turning lack of appetite into such a habit that they become dangerously underweight.

Allergies and sensitivities to wheat, dairy products and gluten products can further complicate nutritional problems. Some dieticians and physicians will test you for substances that may fall within this category if requested. It is not standard in a GP consultation to expect allergen testing, and not all GPs have the time or the facilities. Food sensitivity can be the sole cause of abdominal pain (and sometimes felt in other parts of the body as referred pain), so it is important to rule out allergic responses and sensitivities when you are considering the overview of pain itself.

The book *Healing with Whole Foods* by Paul Pitchford is highly recommended. Pitchford combines Asian traditional cooking with modern nutrition. This book is a standard text for students of acupuncture, whose studies include nutrition as a very important component. Also useful is *The Natural Health Book* by Australian botanist Dorothy Hall.

Vary your dining routine and invite friends over to share meals. You could take it in turns to exchange recipes and to cook. Make any meal a special treat.

Pets as therapy

Just thinking about domestic pets can bring a smile to your face. Certainly small children respond well to pets, as do most adults.

Dear Dogs and Cats

When I say to move, it means go someplace else, not switch positions with each other so there are still two of you in the way.

The dishes with the paw print are yours and contain your food. The other dishes are mine and contain my food. Please note, placing a paw print in the middle of my plate and food does not stake a claim for it becoming your food and dish, nor do I find that aesthetically pleasing in the slightest.

The stairway was not designed by NASCAR and is not a racetrack. Beating me to the bottom is not the object. Tripping me doesn't help, because I fall faster than you can run.

I cannot buy anything bigger than a king-size bed. I am very sorry about this. Do not think I will continue to sleep on the couch to ensure your comfort. Look at videos of dogs and cats sleeping, they can actually curl up in a ball. It is not necessary to sleep perpendicular to each other stretched out to the fullest extent possible. I also know that sticking tails straight out and having tongues hanging out the other end to maximize space used is nothing but sarcasm.

My compact discs are not miniature frisbees.

For the last time, there is not a secret exit from the bathroom. If by some miracle I beat you there and manage to get the door shut, it is not necessary to claw, whine, try to turn the knob or get your paw under the edge and try to pull the door open. I must exit through the same door I entered. In addition, I have been using bathrooms for years and canine or feline attendance is not mandatory.

The proper order is kiss me, then go smell the other dog's butt. I cannot stress this enough. It would be such a simple change for you.

— *Your loving companion*

Many country cottage hospitals and nursing homes worldwide now have a 'pets as therapy' programme where specially trained dogs are welcomed to cheer patients. Some nursing homes and hostels even have resident feline companions highly sought after by those who miss their own.

8

Coping Strategies

Living with pain is nothing if not a challenge. Strategies to help you cope, particularly on the 'hell days' and when problems seem insurmountable, are invaluable. Being prepared for times when you are feeling down, understanding how to conserve your energy and learning how to make the most of your time and strength give you some control over your life, and your pain.

Pacing your activities

One of the most important lessons is 'pacing' and that means measuring out your energy in small doses. Working in a concentrated, uninterrupted way for one hour a day, with the phone on answering machine, door unanswered, visitors told not to call, and not hopping up and down to get the washing done can help you to focus away from your pain on to something productive.

If you do not learn to pace things, you may end up working like crazy one day, because you feel excited about being in less pain, and overdoing it so that the following days are written off and you will not be functioning well at all. So you need to learn your own pace: whatever works for you. Experiment, be brave about this, but don't push yourself. There are times of urgency when you have to perform extra hard but take a rest before your body gives you no choice.

Sufferers of chronic pain may experience occasional great days and the acute pain days may be few and far between. The main thing to keep focusing on, even on your very worst days, is that they will be over soon. It may help to think of them as a wave that will pass. Maybe you will only suffer minutes, perhaps hours, of 'worst' days. But when the pain subsides and life returns to 'normal for you', how relieved and happy you will be. There's nothing like a bout of appalling pain to make you glad for the good days. I wrote this chapter over some particularly bad days when the pain was so great I could only lie on the bed, and to get up and write even one sentence was a labour of love. But I knew I could do it, and I knew things were going to get better. That in itself gave me courage and confidence, and that's important for us all. There will be bad days again, no doubt, but overcoming these periods is something vital to learn.

It is possible to divide bad days into manageable segments. If you are an avid reader, take one page at a time; if a music lover, listen to or play one short piece; when watching television, aim to concentrate from one commercial break to the next.

It is only if you give too much importance to the 'longest day' that it will seem that way — in other words, try not to make too much of it.

You only live one moment at a time, one second even. Don't imagine you will suffer it all at once, and don't presume every second will be equally dreadful. Some of them will be relatively bearable and you'll doze off occasionally if you allow yourself to do so. Meditation, deep breathing, looking at the flowers and plants near to you, stroking your pet, doing anything which is comforting, will make the time pass faster. You can do it.

Here are some additional tips to help you with pacing your day when you have done enough already.

- Don't do anything that does not need doing (which is obvious, but we don't always follow this simple advice).
- Put off phoning others, if this is your usual custom.
- Let someone who cares for you know you are in trouble; delegate when you can.
- Remember talking is exhausting and explaining your symptoms seems to reinforce pain at a time when you want to put it all out of your mind.
- Ask a friend to let someone else know if children must be collected from school or if work must be notified or students postponed — whatever it takes to make your day as simple as possible.

The priority is to get well so you can continue life as you wish to live it, giving when you can and accepting when you cannot.

You probably have a good support system but you may also have a group of people who call on you for help, and sometimes this can be very draining. Explain kindly to those who call on you at such times that you simply are not up to talking to them at this moment. If they are true friends, they will understand. There is no reason to feel bad that you cannot be all things to all who call upon you. It is part of accepting reality to know your limitations and to explain them to those who know and care for you.

As well as pacing, you have to learn to be assertive when necessary. But remember that a polite and considerate patient is going to be much pleasanter for the medical profession to advise, so try to imagine yourself sitting in a busy consulting room if you phone for advice during the day expecting immediate help. Some receptionists assume the dragon-from-hell approach, but many are angels who will find out the information you need and ring back as soon as possible, or you will receive a phone call from the doctor as soon as she is free.

Shifting the focus

Here are some steps you can take when you are feeling down-hearted and dejected.

Practise *not* thinking about yourself and your problems. Start with ten minutes. You may be surprised to realise how self-centred you become when you are in pain or depressed. Increase the time gradually until you have no time to think about yourself other than to do the practical and necessary tasks your energy permits, such as dressing, washing, cooking meals and watering plants. Do them slowly and enjoy the pleasure of each achievement.

Spend more time each day doing things for others. It may be easier to start off with your pet if you have one. (If you haven't, maybe you should consider introducing one into the home — but do not choose a puppy or kitten, which will need too much care and can cause chaos and even damage; a 'pre-loved' animal that needs re-homing and loving rather than toilet training is a better choice.)

Look around and discover the neighbours or friends who may need you to lend them a hand. Possibly you have forgotten you can do this. By this very act you are giving yourself power. You can help others and by so doing gain strength and courage yourself. Looking outwards and away from yourself is like taking a holiday from the problem, and the more you do it the more you lose that self-absorption that increasingly drives others away. Be a survivor and a helper, not a victim.

Stop talking about your illness. If those who love you enquire and expect a reply, tell them briefly but do not repeat yourself. People who care about you naturally want to know how you are progressing or not, as the case may be. However, even if they love you, they do not want a ball-by-ball description of every aspect of the illness.

Involve yourself in some community work. This can be empowering and useful. Apart from helping others, it shifts the focus to the greater universe, a world of much goodness but also of suffering and disillusionment. If you can help just one person a week, you are doing well. Being part of that universe is no longer to be alone.

Smile. Bring your face into that very expression of hope and joy and delight in seeing another person. It does them good and it does you good also.

Keep your mind occupied

There will be times when physical, emotional and chronic pain can be so severe that not only does it totally absorb your very being, but there seems to be nothing you can do to take your mind to a safer place. Probably one of the reasons people turn to complementary and alternative therapy practitioners is because they offer some strategies to cope with this difficult phase of your life.

Meditation techniques can help when you are in such a debilitated state that your body needs total rest from the anguish pain causes. You might learn how to meditate, learning through your very breath control to ease your anguish and pain. An efficient, experienced and empathetic teacher will guide you through the technique and once you are able to do it on your own, or with tapes, even your worst days can be eased substantially by meditation alone.

Some antidepressants are used in the treatment of chronic pain, just as they are for depression, and, when combined with other medication, they have proved to offer relief in many cases.

Belief in your own ability to rescue yourself from the despair of severe pain will give you strength and courage. Even if techniques only last for some fifteen to twenty minutes at a session, this may be sufficient to break that pain cycle and give your body a kick-start back into coping.

Hell days — the ones we'd rather forget

It would be dishonest to pretend you don't have hell days, days when to lift a finger seems too great a challenge. These days happen. It's how you deal with them that matters. The more you prepare on your 'well' days, the better equipped you will be on the 'hell' days.

If you are having a day when the only thing you can do is leave your head on the pillow, make sure you have fluids to drink close at hand. Have a stock of bending straws so you can sip while lying down. Have a supply of sufficient blankets, heaters and hot water bottles to keep you warm — don't be surprised if you suffer from the hots and the colds and be ready to shed layers and add as required. Severe pain really attacks. Don't fight it. Every now and then, and depending on your condition, such days occur. You simply have to obey your body. There is no medal for bravery.

To pretend you don't have bad days leads others who do have them to feel they are a failure. It is not being a failure to listen to your body's warning signs. Pain is a signal that all is not well. You may have brought it on yourself through something unavoidable. It may just be part of the illness to be going through a bad phase, or it may be a new development that you have to adjust to. Your medication may need reviewing or changing. Perhaps you should see the doctor and discuss it, or even make a phone call seeking reassurance. Do not neglect new pain. And when it comes to children and childcare, this medical advice is absolutely vital.

One of the difficult decisions you face is whether to accept the pain as 'par for the course', particularly if you have done something in a different manner, such as lifting a heavy object or walking too far, or performed one of the movements you know exacerbates the pain. Maybe there is some new problem. Most people who suffer from chronic pain are frightened of being hypochondriacs, or of being considered as such. One of my bravest friends neglects her condition occasionally, although she is gravely ill, simply because she does not wish to appear 'attention-seeking'.

For many chronic pain sufferers, simply getting through each day is a minor miracle, particularly if you can do so without complaining or allowing others to be aware of the problem.

For those who live alone, it is good to prepare a list of a few close and true friends who you can call upon in a genuine emergency to do your essential shopping and housework.

If you have a plan in place for your regular needs, such as a cleaner who comes in once a week, you should not need to call upon these friends often. Good friends will always turn their hand to help you, but it is unreasonable to demand frequent help. Let them visit and offer friendship and companionship, but of course you don't want to turn them into servants. Instead, it is better to be aware of the relevant local community services available when you need permanent help. Most local councils and health authorities publish booklets on care for the disabled and frail aged or infirm. If these booklets are not easily found, telephone and ask for one to be sent or enquire at your local health centre or nearest pharmacy. Make sure you already have necessary phone numbers close by for emergency days. Do not be afraid or too proud to ask for help when you really need it.

Talking to a complete stranger, who is trained to do the listening, is often very useful if you are in severe pain. Phone numbers for professional help lines are found at the front of most telephone directories. People who answer the help lines are dedicated and well trained in the skill of listening and also have the knowledge to suggest who else you should contact for further help and advice.

Distraction seems to be one of the best ways of getting through hell days. I always keep at hand my favourite books, videos, musical collection, a radio near my bed and a TV in the bedroom. I can simply lie and allow my body to recuperate while doing as little physical activity as possible.

Sometimes as few as twenty-four hours of almost total bed rest will bring you back to normal. Some doctors discourage this, but on some occasions it is the only solution to make you better so you can function again. Then you can reassess the amount of help you may need and for how many days. If pain is severe (nine on a scale of ten) discuss with a close friend or relative whether this is the time to call in your doctor, or whether they think you should wait until tomorrow to seek medical advice. If your child has pain on a scale of nine, don't ask for another's opinion, just call the doctor.

It ought to go without saying that some symptoms, such as chest pain when combined with changing heart rhythms and arm pain with nausea, should suggest you need to call an ambulance. But if your situation may not seem quite that severe, you may be reluctant to bother the emergency services or be afraid of making a fuss about nothing. Ambulance and emergency services are trained to sort out what is serious and what is not (to 'triage' patients) — that is their job. Probably more trouble is caused by people who don't call the ambulance soon enough than by people who give false alarms.

You or another family member might consider enrolling in a course at St John Ambulance or the Red Cross to learn cardiac pulmonary resuscitation (CPR) and other first aid techniques. It not only teaches you what simple things (and they are simple) to do in an emergency, but will help you recognise what is a serious problem and what is not — knowledge that can help you feel calm and in control. (Every parent should consider doing this during pregnancy as a matter of routine.) Charges are quite reasonable and it is very useful just to know what to do. You may save a life. First aid practices do change, as does equipment, and it is best to be up to date, so it is a good idea to repeat the course every few years.

Putting on a brave face is necessary much of the time. But if you have these terrible hellish days, having a good cry in the privacy of your own bedroom or in the arms of one you love and trust can be very healing: the physical act of crying stimulates the body's natural release of endorphins.

Above all, be kind to yourself. Allow yourself treats, put by a few chocolates or fudge or something that rewards you and comforts you.

Remember your nutrition is especially important on these days. You will probably feel less like preparing meals than at any other time. You may be suffering from nausea (often brought on by severe pain). A useful tip to help the nausea is to have a supply of crystallised ginger in the cupboard at the ready — unless it disagrees with you — as this is perhaps the only anti-nauseant safe for expectant mothers and some pain sufferers find it more satisfactory than some of the anti-nausea medication on prescription.

It's a good idea to stock the freezer with some frozen meals which only need simple heating. And have some homemade or good commercial soups and protein drinks at the ready. Although these foods will not replace good nutrition in the long term, they will guarantee a reliable source of vitamins and minerals and will keep you going for a day or two.

You need plenty of fluids, avoiding coffee and tea (which contain caffeine) as these irritate already inflamed nerves and also strain the kidneys. Drink fruit or herb teas if you like. It is easier to make yourself something you think you might enjoy than to have something just for the sake of it. Bananas and yoghurt are also good standbys. These are all emergency foods to help you get by on a minimum of effort, while providing your body with a source of nutrition.

Add at least one multi-vitamin tablet or capsule, as well as acidophilus bacilli in capsule form. This is to restore good intestinal flora which may be disturbed by antibiotics or nausea and vomiting.

If you are taking antibiotics, remember to leave at least two hours between taking them and the acidophilus, because one affects the power of the other. If your child is the one having the hell day, include one of his favourite foods, even a 'treat', something you usually disallow, unless it is on a banned list for medical reasons.

There is one very definite and comforting thought that you can hold on to: you will never recall the pain exactly as intensely as it was. Otherwise, the human race would have died out a long time ago.

Getting around when you can no longer walk much

All the following information about scooters and wheelchairs is as equally relevant to the needs of children as it is to adults. If their manual dexterity is good, children respond well to learning their use. Being able to join their classmates by bringing their wheelchairs up to the same height level at the push of a button gives them a freedom of which they would otherwise be deprived. And one tip: save up bubble paper and let them ride their motorised vehicle over it as fast as they can do safely. It sounds like a gun popping off and little children adore that — it is important to keep fun in their lives.

If you are able to drive a car, well and good, but only do so on days when pain is not over-riding your judgemental skills and reflexes. If you opt to buy a motorised wheelchair or scooter to give yourself a sense of independence — perhaps to visit neighbours, collect your own post, empty the rubbish, things you used to take for granted — you'll be surprised at the different way people will regard you.

I've tried both options.

A very skilled and kindly scooter salesman — more a social worker at heart I think — brought me four wheelchairs to try in my local shopping centre and left them with me for a whole morning, promising to bring me some scooters in the afternoon. Although I was independent, I did not feel very safe in the wheelchairs, having nothing in front of me and I found them cumbersome to manage in the street going up and down ramps and hills. Later I found a scooter that suited me far better; it has handlebars more like a bicycle.

What was really interesting was the reaction of the public towards me.

The morning wheelchair session took place in the same suburb as the afternoon one and much the same type of people passed by: housewives, young mums, fathers with children in pushchairs and office workers. When I was in a wheelchair they did not greet me, but averted their glance, perhaps assuming I was unable to communicate. However, I received a different response on the cheery red scooter. People stopped to chat, asked me where I got it from, what I used it for, how long I had used one, how much it cost and whether I thought their old mum should get one 'to help her with her independence'. Almost everyone stopped to chat.

Unfortunately, it is difficult to purchase suitable electric wheelchairs or scooters for children as they must usually be custom built and cost almost as much as a brand-new small car, whereas you'll get a suitable range of electric scooters for adults with excellent suspension, lights and horn for about a quarter of that. It's worth getting at least three quotes — after all, every penny counts and being disabled is an expensive business. Ironically, it is hard to sell a second-hand scooter, even at one-quarter of its original price.

I still get frequent requests for the name of my scooter's distributor, multiple questions about how well it does, how far it goes, how much I enjoy it, and so on. It is as if I am a cheerful person who needs a bit of help getting around when I am on a scooter, but in the wheelchair I become one of nature's victims, suffering from some disease that might even be communicable.

Likewise, when I use my manual wheelchair pushed by a friend, she is addressed but people seldom talk to me. I immediately became invisible. It seems there is a public reaction against those in wheelchairs but not against scooter riders. Maybe the scooters are thought of as being more like golf buggies, which suggest health and sportiness — a more favourable image.

It depends on the type of injury you have sustained, or whatever disability or illness you have, which scooter or wheelchair you should choose. It is better to discuss this need with an occupational therapist than with a salesperson, if you are in doubt. I was fortunate in finding a salesman who had a kind honest heart, but few will lend machines on a trial basis. If you have spinal pain, as I do, do not choose a lightweight three-wheel scooter because of their lack of suspension and the quality of footpaths you may have to travel upon. On the three-wheeler, I used to feel as if I had been through a spin-dryer by the time I got home, even from a one-kilometre journey. My new, stronger scooter has full suspension and four wheels and is less likely to tip.

If you cannot afford a new scooter, ask to see second-hand ones. Many are in very good condition and have been used only for a short time. Salespeople will prefer to show you new models, not only for the warranty but of course for the higher commission offered. Buyer beware. And make sure you have it added, complete with serial number, to your household contents insurance — covered against fire and theft, as well as damage to other footpath and road users. This is usually cheaper than taking out a separate policy.

To find outlets selling scooters and wheelchairs, look up

Disability Equipment in the Yellow Pages. You can research types and brands on the internet before you buy. In some jurisdictions, you may be required to register your wheelchair or scooter.

Facing your worst fears

People's worst fears may differ: for some it may be learning they will be unable to walk again or that the pain will never go away, or it may be being told that an illness is terminal. For parents it may be finding out that their child has a life-limiting illness.

Whatever your own worst fears are, they are a challenge and your true and practical self will be discovered. Take your time to make a list of the pros and cons in your life. There will be many of both. Consider all the things you want to do with your nearest and dearest, with your family and friends. Most of your goals will be concerned with people rather than things, on settling old scores, on making peace. If you are in need of help with family conflict resolution, or something has been bothering you which is problematic, please do yourself a favour and sort it out now. The peaceful feeling of resolution will be bound to make you feel better and more able to face your future. You want to leave old baggage behind you — something perhaps you never wished to carry anyway.

And give yourself some treats. You may have always wanted a fountain in your garden. This may seem trivial but if you want it and can afford it, do it. Put one in now. Naturally you must not throw caution to the wind with regard to expense, so discuss the state of your finances with your family. But be wary of giving in to mere expensive whims. You might want to be involved in training guide dogs for the blind, or even some physical feat that involves risk, such as bungee jumping. The list of possibilities is as endless as is the variety of human nature.

If your illness has given you manic strength or obsessive ideas, discuss them with your loved ones. You may discover that illness gives you impulsive enthusiasms and strength that might not last the distance, or obsessive ideas that might not necessarily be the wisest course of action. It is sensible to discuss them carefully.

Simply coping with the reality that you may not survive, and the impact this will have on those who are dear to you, as well as dealing with your own fears, is something for which you may need professional counselling. On the other hand, if you have a strong and reliable sensible support network, discuss things with them. Check the website of Bernie Siegel; his ECaP group accepts emails from all over the world, and advice or group attendance need not cost you money if you don't have it. Siegel lets his facilities and assistance be known, stressing that no one is turned away if they are genuinely in need of help and have no means to pay.

If you are discovering your true self at last, and your ideas are do-able, carry them out. Perhaps you have been a late achiever: now the world is your oyster. From my own experiences, when I might have died and from working with people who have terminal illnesses, I give this advice: put your finances in order and make sure that important things are done. Update your will, discuss it with the person you choose as executor, and think carefully about the effect these decisions will have on those dependent upon you once you have gone. See a good financial advisor you trust or who is recommended by friends, or at least discuss this with your solicitor.

By attending to these matters immediately, and even going so far as planning your funeral music, you are not being morbid, but positive and practical, which will also help those who care for you to cope. If it has not been your habit to talk and discuss important issues previously, this is a great opportunity to start.

When travelling

When travelling overseas or interstate, carry a letter from your physician stating the regular medication you take and what it is for. In certain countries, it is a criminal offence to carry quantities of opiates or opioids, even if they are prescribed, unless you can prove they are for your personal use. Check a relevant government website and register with it after making your travel booking. You will be sent daily updates on dangerous regions and on new terrorist threats and advice on where not to stay. See page 24 for an example of a medical history which includes the type of information you will be expected to provide: major illnesses, surgery, breathing or cardiac problems, allergies and sensitivities, past surgical interventions and in particular clots in the legs (deep vein thrombosis or DVT).

The official government websites will give you advice about travelling overseas with prescription or over-the-counter medications and up-to-date information about recent travel safety changes. These are free services and are invaluable. Don't be surprised by a flood of notifications: you can choose to receive fewer notifications by ticking only the countries you are visiting, and you can un-subscribe at any time.

Check with the same website two weeks prior to departure and again two or three days before leaving, just to double-check information and recent warnings. Also re-confirm flight details, which isn't always easy as all you may get is an answering service. Be persistent if you have special requirements or if you need to speak to a real person.

Although it may not be strictly necessary, it is advisable to carry a letter of clearance for your medication from the embassy or consulate of each country you are visiting. It is important to have this in writing: an email is better than nothing but headed stationery is better still. You can get advice on this from your relevant customs services.

Even with a letter from your doctor, you may still need clearance, and it may save you hours of waiting around. When I travelled to Britain and to France, I got letters from their high commission and embassy respectively, describing the amount of medication I was carrying and needed for six weeks. It may take up to four weeks to get all this done so, unless you are going for an emergency, get your paperwork in order early. It is best to send emails and faxes whenever possible as normal postal services can be delayed. Registered post or express delivery is worth the extra money for the peace of mind it will give you.

The government foreign affairs websites also contain information concerning vaccinations. For example, you may need yellow fever inoculations in certain areas but only if you are coming from specified areas. If your own GP does not have a vaccination service, ask where you can obtain the advice. There are travel clinics in most city centres.

I never risk travelling overseas without a comprehensive health care insurance policy. You may book this through your travel agent or through a firm of your choice; the cheapest option may not be the best one, so ask to see a written policy that shows specific exclusions and inclusions before signing anything. Do not be surprised if pre-existing conditions are excluded, but don't despair if this is the case because often you will be able to pay a reasonable premium to have these included, at least for emergency care.

You cannot rely on your country's embassy in the region to which you are going as your only backstop: there may be another more pressing emergency such as the recent hurricanes and earthquakes which overextend their services. There are some sensible precautions to take:

- Keep a copy of your passport, vaccination certificates, travel documents (including doctor's letter) and birth certificate on a friend's computer so these details can be faxed or emailed through. Make sure that the friend is not going to be away at any date during your absence; it is probably worth giving a second person the details too. Or email them to yourself — you can pick up messages at internet cafés.

- Keep several copies of the above in easily accessible places: in your hand luggage, handbag or briefcase and in your checked-in baggage.

Ensure you pack your luggage yourself. Customs officials will ask you to sign a document to this effect. This is especially important if you are carrying proscribed or restricted medicines such as opioids.

These are sensible precautions for those who do require substantial quantities of medication, particularly opioids. Even codeine (which you may consider a harmless over-the-counter tablet yet is derived from the opiate family) is banned in certain countries.

Drinking alcohol while flying in the already over-dry atmosphere further dehydrates your body, possibly causing more jet lag during and after the flight, which can worsen your pain. This doesn't mean you should not have a glass of wine with your meal, but don't overdo the free champagne just because you are travelling first or business class.

Travelling like a sardine in a tin is uncomfortable anyway, and if you can possibly afford an upgrade it is worth it, particularly if you suffer from back pain — as the seat size in economy class is miserly. Airline websites will give information on the exact sizes, dimensions and slant of seats if your travel agent is unable to or unwilling to check it for you. Also search for comments from travellers on the internet to compare with the airlines' own sometimes exaggerated claims of 'luxury' and comfort. Travelling long haul can seldom be truly comfortable, even in first class.

I once travelled with a full bottle of liquid morphine sulphate in my handbag. On descent to Singapore airport, a sudden change in air pressure caused the glass bottle, hitherto unopened, to explode. I was carrying this medicine legally and possessed various copies of doctors' letters (which was just as well, as it turned out). My passport and travel documents, the all-important doctor's permit, plus earplugs, handkerchiefs and combs ended up covered in a sloppy mess of sticky fluid. Since all the toilets seemed occupied, I buzzed for the stewardess and cautiously asked if I might 'use the kitchen sink to dispose of some liquid spilled in my bag'. Not unreasonably, she offered to do this for me, but I declined (I had signed a document promising to keep control of my opioids at all times) and said I would prefer to do it myself. 'What is it that I cannot pour down the sink, then?' she asked. I replied calmly, 'Look, it's only morphine.' A little shaken, she escorted me to the sink and helped wipe down my sodden documents and passport, although she did summon another stewardess to witness what was occurring. (If you do carry liquid medicine in your handbag, open the bottle before you leave and allow some air in, then take the precaution of wrapping the bottle in plastic secured with elastic bands.)

On arrival, I was escorted by a guard, but he was a pleasant young man employed to look after wheelies. The Customs official looked at my sodden letter as one would at excrement, waved me through and I was free to go to my hotel. But it was a very tense situation.

One more point about travelling: the carriage of wheelchairs and or invalid scooters. You must declare that you are taking a wheelchair or scooter with you when you book — you may be asked for the height, width and weight of your vehicle so have this information readily to hand. Most airlines carry the vehicles free of charge and do not weigh them or charge you with excess baggage. If the person at the check-in desk tries to do this, ask to see the supervisor and explain that you have been informed that the airline does not make a charge for this service (but make sure of this when you book your ticket). The details of your wheel-chair or scooter should be on the airline's computer. If you have been unlucky enough to have chosen one of the few airlines that does charge, hopefully you will have been told in advance and have had time to appeal against this (in most cases, charges are waived). Know your rights, particularly if you are travelling to a country where you do not know the language. If you need an interpreter when encountering a difficult situation, ask for one.

If you are taking a battery-operated wheelchair or scooter, you will have to make sure the type of battery is suitable for air travel (best done when you purchase the machine, if you travel frequently). You may be asked to separate the batteries and have them specially wrapped when checking in, and will be given an airport wheelchair and allocated a porter who will accompany you right up to the aircraft door. Usually this speeds you through Customs. The normal drill is, wheelies on first and off last. If you tell those meeting you at the airport that you may be delayed up to half an hour while this happens, they will not worry when they see everyone else coming out first.

Also, it is a wise precaution to arrive at the airport check-in at least half an hour earlier than suggested on your ticket so that formalities concerned with the comfort of your journey to the plane and arrangements about your chair can be made easily. Try to avoid creating emergency situations, take a good book and be prepared for a long wait.

If you are travelling business or first class, you may be taken to a special lounge where you will be more comfortable during the inevitable waits. There are usually showers and sometimes saunas and massage rooms available for your use as well as snacks, free tea and coffee or alcoholic beverages.

Also, a tip that has worked for me: you are more likely to be given an up-grade (free of charge) if you are smartly dressed. This is prejudice again on dress code, especially as many business–class travellers carry a comfy track suit to change into prior to boarding or on the plane itself. Loose fitting clothing is important for comfort but that doesn't mean you need to be sloppily dressed.

Your comfort, particularly on a long-haul flight, will greatly influence the amount of pain you suffer in transit. All planes carry oxygen supplies, and if you are anxious or in pain, ask the on-board crew if you could have some oxygen for your condition (without causing panic among other passengers). I've always found airline crews are most willing to help, to give you an extra blanket if you are chilly, and pillows to prop you into a better position.

If you dehydrate quickly, always carry a water bottle. A litre in a plastic bottle in your hand luggage will make the difference between dry mouth misery and comfort and will mean you always have a supply when you need to take your medication.

My son, who makes approximately twenty long-haul world journeys per annum in his work, has the following tips:

- No alcohol.
- Carry at least one litre of water.
- Carry a packet of plain sweet biscuits.

- Ask for vegetarian meals when you make your booking (these are less likely to contain rich, indigestible food).
- If you have special dietary requirements, state them when you book, or at least two weeks' prior to departure.
- Wear an eye mask and use your ear plugs.
- Tell the crew not to wake you when you are asleep (American airlines apparently wake everyone anyway).
- Don't start a conversation with those sitting next to you if you want to sleep.

9

Children with Pain

It is difficult enough just being a parent. But it can be very frightening when your children or those in your care are sick. Looking after anybody with a serious illness is a big responsibility and you need the help of experts.

In today's world, where possibly both parents work, children often feel second-best and less important than 'Mummy or Daddy's work' — so just by showing them that you can put them first will give them comfort and may help get them over an episode which could otherwise grow into a much more serious problem.

Some employers are very reasonable about allowing parents compassionate leave when they have a sick child, and the only certificate a doctor need write is one which indicates that 'the parent is unable to attend work because of their child's unfitness for school'. Working mothers in particular often feel sufficient guilt as it is, without making them feel a failure at work as well as at home.

Believing your child

Listening carefully to what children and their families say about their pain is a vital part of understanding the needs of the individual child and is an essential part of holistic and comprehensive nursing care. As an adult you will know how threatening it feels when your medical practitioner fails to believe in your pain. Alas, this is very common, particularly with persistent pain that cannot be measured effectively by data, procedures or hard evidence.

You know your child better than the nurses and the doctors do. It is important for you to build a good relationship with your treating physicians and nurses so that they believe you, as you are the advocate for your child's needs.

When your child suffers from chronic or recurring pain, it is important to seek medical intervention as soon as possible so that the cause is correctly diagnosed. As episodes of pain vary so much both in length and intensity, and can be brought on by factors including stress, be watchful to ensure the pain is not exacerbated by changes and pressures at home and at school. These episodes of pain can be set off by the awareness of tensions within the home, when parents may be on the verge of separating or divorcing, when a family member or close friend has died or is dying, or merely by a change of house or school, which can be quite traumatic to a child who is only just coping on a day-to-day basis anyway because of an underlying illness.

Generally you will know if the child is 'putting it on'. But sometimes you won't. Unless your child has a particularly strong history of hypochondriacal behaviour or of avoidance of school, there will be an underlying reason for this. Is your child being bullied? Are you having trouble in your relationships at home? Is there a new baby who has replaced the child's starring order in the household? These types of factors may be behind your child's reporting of pain. Sometimes psychiatric or psychological counselling will be required.

It is important to recognise that psychological causes of pain syndromes are diagnosed when there is clear evidence for them, and it is not just as a diagnosis of convenience. At most clinics where such testing, monitoring and counselling is done, physical causes of illness are ruled out before it is assumed that the child requires psychological help.

Effective pain management starts with a commitment to believe in the pain that the child is reporting and working with him and his family to achieve the best control possible. Pain is a problem in its own right.

In western culture, pain is often seen as being synonymous with wrongdoing and punishment, and this often makes pain harder to bear, especially for a child. Religious teaching and a belief in 'karma' can lead adults to believe their child's pain is due to something she has done for which she is now being punished. Fortunately, such erroneous and punitive thinking no longer occurs in most families. Not long ago, the bedwetting child would have been put in a cold bath all night to cure him of his 'evil doing', and this by god-fearing parents who did it for the 'good of the child'. This occurred in families as recently as the late 1950s when I was working in the Child Guidance Clinic at Oxford. Naturally, this cruel punishment caused additional problems, often leading to urinary tract infections, chills and stomach and back pain. Psychologically, the damage would cause further fear and forever associate enuresis (bedwetting) with punishment and guilt. This practice was common in institutional care, particularly that undertaken by some of the religious orders. Fortunately this rarely happens today.

The most obvious person to ask about the level and type of pain is the sufferer and, in the case of childhood pain, this is something that is not done frequently enough. There are some inherent difficulties in getting this information from children, especially young ones. But that is no excuse for not trying and there are some effective techniques. When I was interviewing a seven-year-old in hospital about his pain and what he thought could be its cause, he looked me straight in the eye and sighed heavily and then he said, 'Pain hurts, stupid.' Good for him.

You can encourage the child to communicate the quality of her pain by the use of drawings. This can be a powerful way of demonstrating the impact that pain has on her life. Sand play has long been used under the supervision of psychotherapists and reveals family relationship imbalances, perceptions of neglect, real or imagined. If what it reveals makes sense to you, take steps to make your child happier. If the opinion given by the therapist seems of little value, and not evidence-based, or you doubt the therapist's qualifications, seek another opinion.

Pain is often an all-consuming experience for the child and one that he often finds difficult to explain to adults. Recurrent severe pain over a prolonged period is much more significant and serious than people realise in that it exhausts the sufferer and diminishes his quality of life.

Most major pain episodes are self-contained and predictable and the child is pain-free between episodes — for example, as in recurrent ear infections, irritable colon and bowel disease. Very often, allowing a child 'time out' at home with a caring parent, friend or grandparent can remove some of the stress that may be exacerbating pain that is not serious. Irritable colon is a good example of the benefits of allowing the child time off and bed rest, tucked up warmly with a hot water bottle, a favourite toy and the domestic pet, with mum, dad or a loved and trusted family friend at home making special time for the child.

Going to the doctor

As discussed earlier, communication with a medical practitioner is not always easy. It may be even harder to act as the spokesperson for one of your children.

The relationship you build with your doctor is vital. As the advocate for your child, finding the right doctor is imperative. If you are fortunate and happy with your GP, you can stay with her for most of your family's needs. She in turn will recommend a suitable paediatrician or specialist when this is appropriate.

You will need to focus on the information you require before you go to an appointment. If your child is over the age of four, he will be able to tell you things he wants to ask, but he will probably need some prompting.

The following are 'analysed consultations', which show some of the issues that might arise in interactions with a health professional, in this case a doctor.

Why not begin by saying to your child: 'We're going to see a new doctor on Friday, and I have a few questions I want to ask her about helping your pain. What would you like to ask? I'll write down your questions on my pad beside the questions I want to ask.'

By framing your words this way your child feels he has control over the situation. It is his pain after all. Prompt him if he can't explain himself easily. Many children enjoy play-acting: you can pretend to be the doctor and assume a different voice, maybe examine him, and let him explain in his own words what the problem is. Help him to feel confident about explaining it.

Unfamiliar consulting rooms may be worrying for your child, so prepare him for the visit, and maybe take along one of his favourite books or toys. Depending on their age, children sometimes like to show the doctor where teddy suffers pain rather than to show their own body initially. On a first visit, he may be curious or concerned and anxious. (Recently I watched a little girl of four go into a hairdresser's with her mother. She had been playing happily with her doll outside the shop, but the moment she went in and sat in the chair waiting for her hair to be cut, she began the most frightful screaming fit. She was placated by the offer of a bottle of water to squirt at the hairdresser, a useful distraction.)

Bring the list of the questions you want to ask with you to the consulation. Have a copy for the doctor and hand it to her with a smile. Introduce the problem and explain why you like to write the questions down. This gives the doctor time to assess more about you. She may be grateful that you expect the session to be structured. Many of us become confused and then distracted from the main points of the consultation, and this can be tiresome for the doctor and time-wasting.

For example, a mother is taking her five-year-old son Paul, who has been suffering excruciating head pains for two weeks, to see a paediatrician recommended by the family doctor. This is the first appointment. To date, the headaches had been treated, on the GP's advice, with paracetamol.

'We really need your help to manage Paul's pain,' the mother says. 'We are not coping well on our own. Here are some of the things that are happening. Paul is unable to sleep through the night. He wakes with pain at least four times. He complains of nightmares, frequently wets the bed, and asks to sleep in our bed, with me and his father. If his medication is not due, can I give him an extra dose then, or must I wait till the morning?'

Use a friendly and positive voice, and allow time for your doctor to respond rather than reeling off a long speech. It's unreasonable to expect the doctor to remember your every word. Also, she may need to get a lot more information from you and Paul before she can come back to your question. Although you are the advocate for your child, don't be surprised if the doctor will want to ask your child's opinion and will need to hear the way he explains his pain.

She might turn to Paul to ask him about his pain and his trouble at night. Paul may say, 'I get so sleepy at school because I don't sleep at night. And then this pounding starts in my head and I can't pay attention.' It's important that Paul has the chance of bringing up the 'pounding'. It may indicate some important symptom the doctor wants to check.

However, your observations are important too. You might explain, 'During the day Paul has temper tantrums which can last for thirty or forty minutes and I can't handle these. He clutches at his head with pain and screams at me when I try to calm and cuddle him. Is there anything you can give him to calm him down and can I give him an additional dose if the first one doesn't work?'

The doctor might have to ask a lot more questions of you, or Paul, before she can answer that.

Paul may say, 'Doctor, when my head hurts, it feels like an exploding balloon.' To the doctor, it means much more if the child uses his own words. The doctor can formulate questions accordingly, asking exactly where the balloons are and how often they explode, for example.

If you have the impression that the doctor is not really listening to you or your child, if she appears preoccupied or perhaps allows constant interruptions with phone calls, speak up but always be respectful. You might like to make these points: 'Doctor, I'm really anxious about Paul and I need this time with you. Would it be possible to divert phone calls during our consultation? Watching Paul fidget, I know it distresses him too. I worry we are going to run out of time before we have had a chance for you to help us.'

State exactly what you mean. If you don't think you've said it clearly or if you feel you've been misunderstood, rephrase your questions. Once again, allow the doctor time to reply. Doctors are just as likely to suffer from headaches, bad tempers, days when they are not communicating well, just as we do. But although you can make allowances for this, realise how vital this association is and follow your instinct. She may apologise and explain that there is some particular call she is waiting for which is very important to the safety of another patient. If no satisfactory explanation is offered, be on your guard.

Occasionally you may be unlucky in your choice of doctor, and it is your right to seek the best medical opinion available. If you don't make a good connection with the doctor or feel she dislikes or misunderstands you, it is best to find someone with whom you are happier. It is easy to get things wrong when you are upset and anxious, and it may be a good idea to plan several visits before making a definitive decision if you think you need a change.

But let's imagine you ask, 'My husband is getting very angry at the loss of sleep at night. Can you help him to get back to sleep by prescribing sleeping pills for him?' The doctor is seeing you about your son, not about your husband, and this is not the right time to bring up such an issue. The doctor almost certainly won't write a prescription for your husband, and you must accept her decision. Just as you expect the doctor to do her best by you, she expects you to follow her advice. It is a contract of trust.

If medication is prescribed for your child, you might want to ask, 'Can you explain how it works and what we can expect? So far, with the paracetamol, Paul seems to be getting worse rather than better.' Pause again to allow the doctor time to answer. By showing that you are listening to her, you are encouraging her to listen to you too.

The doctor might suggest some new medication for Paul. It

is reasonable to ask, 'Will there be any side effects? If so, how will I know which ones are serious?'

The doctor may give you a list or show you a leaflet describing the medication. She may, for example, explain that Paul might suffer from dry mouth, drowsiness or dizziness. She should tell you which of these symptoms will be unimportant or will lessen in time, and explain what to do if there is a more serious problem.

It is so important to clear up any questions about side effects at the consultation, so that you leave the doctor's rooms with confidence that you understand the medication prescribed and its uses, its advantages and possible disadvantages. There are very few magic bullets. Almost every medicine has some possible side effects — if it doesn't, it probably doesn't work at all. Deciding to use it is about weighing up the pros and cons, and it's good to get some idea of how the doctor is thinking. Also being aware of minor side effects can help prevent later anxiety that can undermine your trust in the doctor.

A pitfall can be those lists of possible side effects produced by the pharmaceutical companies to protect themselves. On the one hand, the drug companies always insist that a medicine is safe; on the other hand, they produce a list that would terrify anyone who reads it. During the drug's research period, any side effect must be reported and the patient making the report may exaggerate the effect, so do not be over-anxious about these lists. Listen to what your doctor has to say instead. Luckily, you will read about the side effects on behalf of your child, who won't be prejudiced into imaginary symptoms, but you will know what to look out for.

The doctor may recommend tricyclic antidepressants in the treatment of certain types of pain. This may prompt you to declare, 'But none of Paul's behaviour suggests that he is depressed or sad.' Although this may well be the case, chronic pain can, of itself, cause a form of depression simply in the way it prevents the patient (of any age) from leading the life formerly enjoyed.

Another medication you may be given for the condition could be an anti-epileptic preparation. Once again you may protest, 'But Paul is not an epileptic.' The doctor can tell you how the medication helps alleviate pain and spasms in certain types of conditions and further explain the reasons for its use.

It is a good idea while you are at the consultation to write down the doctor's advice concerning dosages, particularly when you must build up from a low to a higher dose, and the time between doses, so you can note these changes in your diary or on the kitchen calendar. There is so much to remember from a consultation that you will get the greatest benefit from it if you have taken notes that you can use as a reminder. (If doses do have to be increased over time, your pharmacist may well be happy to make up a tray of doses in special containers with times and days marked on them.)

The important thing is to establish dialogue, to gain confidence and to ask appropriate questions. As Paul is five years old, he will need help but will be able to express himself. With a younger and/or less verbal child, of course, you must formulate the questions. An infant or toddler will need you to do almost all the talking, but older children might have their questions for the doctor, and may need your help in how to voice them.

Older children

Amanda is eleven years old, and has been having painful heavy periods for the past six months. She is embarrassed at school with flooding and, as the periods are irregular, is often unprepared. You discuss the matter initially with your family doctor, the man who has been treating you all for ages, but she refuses to see a male doctor. He refers her to a friendly female gynaecologist in whom he has every confidence. Even then, Amanda tells you she doesn't like the idea of being examined. You discuss this with her and suggest she writes her questions down.

Teenagers are often uncomfortable with their body image and ill at ease with physical examinations. As a parent, help them with this and accompany them to the doctor's if they want you to. Equally, they may prefer you to come to their appointments with them and wait outside the consultation room. Fourteen-year-old Gregory was sent home from school with severe pain in his side. He didn't want his mother to come in to see the GP with him, but was grateful she was there when, after examination, he was diagnosed with an inflamed appendix and immediate admission to hospital was arranged.

Procedures and treatments

When your child is undergoing painful or uncomfortable procedures and treatments, you will want to be there to provide support, and distraction if possible.

One form of distraction could be music therapy where the child is actively engaged in learning a simple tune and playing it on an instrument (such as a guitar or drum, or maracas made from empty plastic bottles with dry rice or pasta inside) while supervised by a music therapist, who could ask the child to compose words describing his pain. They might then sing a song together to a well-known tune, something easy they can remember. Many of the children (aged ten to twelve) at one particular hospital composed complex words to describe the isolation of pain, as much as its severity. Any form of distraction involving the attention of the patient may well help with pain relief.

Try to engage yourself in the activity with the child (hide any tears — make a quick toilet visit, if necessary) and do your best to remain bright and cheerful because this, of itself, gives the child strength and courage, just seeing that you are not upset (and in turn you will gain confidence too). It's difficult to remain cheerful and positive when your child is having repeated procedures, such as failed venipuncture attempts, but perhaps telling stories they love, playing a tune for them on an iPod close to their ear or just holding a hand may assist with pain relief. It's all part of the good parenting you probably do instinctively anyway.

In various surveys, parents were asked if they would consider reassurance or distraction to be the most effective way to quell a child's anxiety prior to painful procedures. Most said that distraction was the best therapy, and indeed it is in most circumstances. Naturally, reassurance is necessary but it is not sufficient. It is of little comfort to say 'Mummy is here and nothing which is going to happen will hurt', because lumbar punctures are painful unless local anaesthetics (injection or gel) are given first. Your child will feel betrayed if you lie about this.

Be there, and hold your child's hand by all means, but take along a favourite book or involve her in a story, something she knows by heart or make one up on the spot and work on it together, including ridiculous and humorous vocabulary to truly distract. Blowing bubbles is useful too but not always possible — it depends on the procedure. Simply being aware of doing these helpful, distracting things will reassure you also, as an anxious parent. If possible, keep your anxiety and tears away from your child's sight. If you need to cry, hug your child, make sure a nurse or care worker stays with her, and go somewhere private to do your weeping.

You are expected to be the strong one, even if you feel that you are dying inside. Be there as the strong protective guardian of your child's life. Knowing how important this is to your child will, of itself, help you to be strong and keep your mind on the main purpose, which is to make your child feel less afraid.

Managing pain at school

If it is possible for your child to keep going to school, you will need to make sure the teachers understand the nature of her illness and what special needs she may have. It is amazing how groups of children adapt to the needs of a child within their group, treating any special equipment (wheelchairs, respirators, oxygen tanks) as a normal part of living. If school teachers are well prepared, they will welcome her back into their midst and ease the problems of missed schooling. A wise teacher will recruit classmates into her care in small ways. They might advise the class to avoid bumping her if the source of her pain is musculoskeletal, and appoint a special 'chum' within the class who will keep an eye on her and help her if she is experiencing difficulties in mobility or management of tasks. The teachers must treat the child positively and do all that is possible to include her in normal activities so she feels integrated and part of her former group.

Severe or new symptoms: going to hospital

There will be days, those hell days for parents, when watching a child suffering pain is so unbearable we wish we could take the pain and suffer it for them.

If your child suffers from severe abdominal pain, make sure you do not administer food or drink, for should there be an obstruction, inflammation or appendicitis, fasting is required prior to emergency admission for surgery. One of the reasons for this is that a prescribed length of time is necessary prior to an anaesthetic being administered as this helps to eliminate the likelihood of vomiting.

When you telephone the doctor, give the case history and symptoms clearly, noting the onset of pain, foods that have been eaten recently or whether another family member has similar symptoms (it might be food poisoning). The GP may make a home visit or arrange for an admission to hospital by ambulance, as he sees fit.

If you have to call an ambulance, make sure the hallway entrance is free from obstructions, as the officers may need to bring in a stretcher. You may need to give them the child's history again as they may not have been given full information by the switchboard operator. If a child has been vomiting or unable to retain food or drink for over twenty-four hours, the crew may attempt to put in a canula for an intravenous drip and commence re-hydration. As this procedure can be painful, an expert may be needed, in which case, the paramedics may await arrival at hospital.

One new practice in France is for the ambulance officer to give the child a furry hand puppet, which is used to find out how much pain the child is suffering from. The child is given ten large tokens (large enough so they can't be swallowed) and asked to give the puppet as many tokens as is necessary to calm the pain represented. On discharge from hospital the child is allowed to keep the soft toy that has kept her company in hospital.

If the doctor in accident and emergency is unable to insert the canula, an anaesthetist will usually be called. Insertion of canulas can be particularly painful for children with very small veins. If you see your child is suffering from too many attempts, insist on a pause and ask if some anaesthetic cream may be applied to the arm. Although this takes up to ninety minutes to be fully effective, it may save the child much pain and trauma during the procedure and subsequently.

You'll have your own special ways to comfort and distract your child. You can use stories, songs or create a diversional activity which is appropriate and in which the child can participate. Blow bubbles if you have any with you. Play 'voices' with a favourite teddy, and encourage the child to describe what is happening to teddy, as if teddy is the patient.

Above all, show confidence rather than fear, even if you are feeling very emotional and fearful. To see you sitting calmly is much more comforting for your child than if you are teary-eyed and begging for the reassurance of the treating doctors and nurses.

Staying in hospital

When you go to the hospital to visit your child, bring her some items that she might miss, such as some recently taken photos of the family on an excursion or of the family cat, a painting done in school, some craft work, a favourite game to share. Obviously this selection will depend not only on the age of the sick child but on the medical condition and length of hospital stay.

When your child is in hospital, the whole family is involved. This may be one of the most anxious times of your life. You should also be aware that your other children will be affected, both emotionally and practically, by the illness. Additional pressures at home can be avoided by good planning. The organisation of practical matters helps the mind to focus away, briefly at least, from worrying about the sick child. It really will help to establish clear guidelines for routines at home so that siblings and parents can each manage hospital visiting, as well as allowing life to continue as closely as possible to that which you enjoyed prior to illness.

It is an unfortunate fact that much of the practice carried out in hospitals is organised by administrators with rule books and little recognition of the effect their ideas may have on the children, and seldom with reference to the nursing unit manager or paediatricians. An arbitrary age may be set, say sixteen, when a child suddenly is deemed to be an adult. His illness, painful condition and symptoms are exactly as they were the day he was fifteen years and 364 days; however, he is expected to adjust to the change from the cushioned care of a paediatric department (which, in some ways, may also be difficult for the mature child to remain in) to an adult unit and expected to interact with adults without the soft lights, music therapy, starlight reviews, teddy bears or the other things that made him feel secure at the children's hospital. The transition is forced upon him when he may not be ready. Both boys and girls are equally affected and, although girls may mature more easily and be more ready, it depends on the individual.

Many paediatricians will ask for special arrangements to be made only to find the hospital rules or the health funding requirements do not allow a person over sixteen to remain in paediatric care. There does have to be a cut-off point, but the child must be eased into it gently, with special care and common sense. The latter is not always the case, alas. Time and funding are often given as very real excuses why the child must move, but at least the parents should be made aware of the difficulties so they can inform themselves through reading and discussion. This is where some self-help groups are invaluable. Ask your child's consultant or your GP for recommendations.

Suzy's story

In April 2005, the *Sydney Morning Herald* reported how difficult it is for young chronic pain sufferers who have been 'nursed' through the paediatric hospital system until their late teens and then moved to an adult ward, where they are then responsible for their own medication, medical history and recording their allergies, and do not often have their parents present. It is a big leap for them, and causes much tension and anxiety. A gradual progression with an explanation from the medical team who have hitherto treated them would help them to move from the adolescent to the adult hospital care.

I interviewed Suzy in hospital at the request of her treating physician. Suzy falls between the paediatric and adult age, and has been permitted to attend an adult facility. But, by having her own room, she is cushioned from the harsher aspects of adult hospital admissions as opposed to the softer life in a paediatric ward. She is sixteen years old.

Some of the points Suzy wanted to make are universal and very helpful. She has been suffering chronic pain and repetitive strain injury from playing her cello over ten years. As a talented prodigy, this has been a depressing and life-changing experience for her. She can only practise the cello for up to twenty minutes each session, two or three times on a good day, which she experiences but a few times each week. She is able to describe her condition, its management and her relationship with her siblings, the hospital staff and her school. She suffers a great deal uncomplainingly but what she says is important to note and may be affecting other children who suffer chronic pain or similar distress.

Top of her list of complaints is that nurses fail to give the correct dose of opioids. Opioids would not generally be required or prescribed for repetitive strain injury, but due to her allergic reaction to medication previously prescribed, after many trials this was found to be the only suitable medication to relieve her intense pain. Many of the nurses failed to understand this and, without checking the doctors' orders, they made her feel guilty for needing a relatively high dose.

She was particularly upset that one nurse told her that an adult suffering from a broken hip 'did not need as much pain relief as you are having', which was said in an accusatory manner. This indicates the need for nurses and medical students to be taught the importance not only of following the instructions of specialists but to understand the use of opioids in the treatment of chronic pain.

She reported that her current dose of Capanol (an opiate derivative) is 270 milligrams per day, in addition to Neurontin (an anti-epileptic drug used in treatment of pain without the presence of epileptic symptoms), which eases her spasms.

With considerable insight, she discussed her medication. Initially, Suzy told me, she had been averse to accepting opioids for pain relief as she had witnessed the extreme mood swings in her sister (who suffered from a similar syndrome) and did not wish to be as difficult a family member as her sister had been. This she reported with compassion and understanding. She said that she was frightened of the possibility of 'addiction', but her doctor had explained that if she were given the dose at the level to relieve pain only, and she never experienced a 'high', her risk of addiction was lessened, and that the dose had been measured specially for her by a pain specialist who knew her case and her symptoms and who visited her every day to monitor her progress. The combination of opiates with other tablets had caused adverse reactions. She reported that Tramol (another medication offering opiate-like pain relief) had given her such adverse reactions that she developed a syndrome resulting in a tremor of some severity. Suzy was able to laugh when I suggested this would have helped with her vibrato, and was able to relate to the funny side of things very well.

Her recent hospital admission followed a bad reaction to a cortisone injection. Normally, she says, her pain is at a level of around four to six. However, on admission she was up to a ten, the worst pain she had ever experienced.

Suzy has developed a great sensitivity to the needs and feelings of her siblings and says that one of her brothers is very tender and exceptionally understanding for a boy of fifteen. We agreed, jokingly, that particularly at this age, boys can be 'a bit of a problem'.

At home she did have a maternal model of injury as her mother had suffered a work-related RSI-type neck injury, which had required six weeks of hospitalisation and resulted in her requiring opioids to manage the ongoing pain.

Once more, Suzy stated that to 'use' opioids was against her wishes initially. I suggested she substitute the word 'use' with the simple one 'take' and instead of 'drugs' say 'medication', which would make it easier to explain to her friends that she required medicine to help her to function. She thought about this and said one of the sad things is explaining to her peers why she requires a nebuliser (for asthma), so she was beginning to feel like a 'weirdo' anyway. Now that she also had to take so many tablets just to keep functioning, we agreed this was a time she would discover true friendship and solidarity. She seemed cheered when I told her I require opioid medication to function — she found great relief in that.

She says, with some pride, that her family is very close and united, that their musical activities give them much joy and that they will continue to book tickets to musical events, which boosts her spirits even if she is ill and unable to attend some performances because of pain.

Suzy listed the most distressing thoughts concerning her illness: Why did this happen to me? What have I done to deserve this? Why do I always end up missing the most important things because I fall ill?

She is an exceptionally gifted child who comes across, on first meeting, as sad but without self-pity and wise beyond her years. As a keen musician, she had been practising seven hours a day and taking private lessons in piano, clarinet and cello. Due to her severe asthmatic condition, she had not been admitted to a top music school, which lacks the facilities to care for someone with such a condition. Instead, her education is conducted via the Correspondence School. Although this keeps her up-to-date with her studies, it does deprive her of the companionship of her peers and she experiences loneliness and isolation because of this. Were her family not so supportive, her life would be considerably less bearable.

Among the measures that were taken to help Suzy was her gradual part-time admission to the local high school, with the teachers and class made aware of the extreme circumstances of her illness and occasional inability to attend or to perform homework. This had been discussed with the local head teacher, who agreed to limit her attendance to three mornings a week, to support her personally, to ensure her medicine is taken at the right time and, in an emergency, to refer her back to the pain clinic for admission as required.

Several months after our initial interview, Suzy reported that the inclusion in class lessons had cheered her spirits, she had given a talk on chronic pain to a school assembly and was comforted by the support of teachers and fellow students. She expressed gratitude that things were beginning to work well for her. She was even considering joining the school orchestra.

From Suzy we can learn that a positive attitude, an understanding of her condition (by Suzy and those around her) and an organised, paced schedule with her music acting as a distraction when she is well enough to participate, plus strong family support, have been of great help to her.

Interview with John's mother

John is a country child living in New South Wales. His journey time to the main children's facility is around ninety minutes. John's mother can imagine how difficult it must be for country parents who live even further away from a major hospital. His parents take it in turns to stay at home with John, and this is difficult for them financially. Heavy costs are involved and the other children often feel left out of the equation.

I met John's father by chance and he told me his son was suffering great pain. I interviewed John's mother by email and then followed it up by telephone.

What did you know about your child's illness when you first came to see the doctor?

This is a bit hard to answer but we were first told John had major congenital heart disease when he was six weeks old. So many other problems and diseases have been diagnosed over the four years since then: congenital heart disease — John has had multiple surgery to repair these problems and will require further operations, but when is not yet known: Hirschsprung's disease — following many bowel operations and obstructions, he now has a permanent colostomy; a severe feeding problem with reflux — John has had a gastrostomy tube since age one; microcephaly (a head and brain much smaller than considered normal) with severe developmental delay; also epilepsy, immune deficiency, severe ear problems with chronic infections needing 'grommets' and kidney reflux.

Did you feel confident that you would be able to explain these procedures to your child?

No, due to his developmental delay he just knows hospital means 'pain' and sometimes separation from his family.

When you were concerned about the pain your child might suffer or was already suffering, were you worried about how you would cope with helping him?

A very big yes!

What would you like to see available to help you cope with this and future health problems in your family?

Maybe a pain management consultation before an operation or a long hospital stay would help. I think, however, that many doctors and nurses dismiss a disabled child's cries, moans and self-harming acts as a 'behaviour problem' rather than accepting the obvious: that the child is in pain and those family members who live with and dearly love that child understand and have learned how their own child shows signs of 'pain'.

Do you use the internet to find answers to your questions or does this baffle you?
Sometimes, but I have not found any great help with it. I do belong to a G-tube chat room, mostly parents from USA, and I have found some answers to tube-feeding problems there.

If you had to choose between reassuring him or distracting him when a procedure is being performed, which would you assume would help him most?
In John's case 'distraction' is the way to go. [Ten out of twelve parents interviewed agreed, and this is certainly the finding of epidemiological study groups.]

Do you like to be present at procedures? If not, what troubles you most?
Most procedures when possible, because we can sing to John and use other forms of distraction and this always makes the procedure easier for him and for doctors and nurses.

Are there things you would like to see changed for children receiving treatment to make the situation easier?
Some situations of course I would love to change but in reality

just more understanding from certain staff members (although a lot are great). Some could do with a large dose of 'compassion' and understanding and insight into the long-term suffering a child with such problems and his family have already been through. They should also be aware of all further reactions to treatments and illnesses.

Are you comfortable discussing problems with the therapeutic team?
Sometimes, but a therapeutic 'team' is hard to come by.

How do you involve the other children in the family with care for John when he is sick?
They are both involved in John's care in some way ... my husband works at night so often my thirteen-year-old will need to help me in physical care, but I try and let them just 'play' with him. My three-year-old keeps asking, 'When will John walk and talk?' And this can be hard to explain.

Is it sometimes impossible for you or your husband to come to the hospital together, and if so, who do you entrust to spend time with him?
There are only a few people who are able to look after John and they can only do some of his care, so we can never leave him for any length of time. Those people include my mum (she lives six hours away) who is a registered nurse. A couple of paid home-care workers care for him for periods of four to eight hours.

What is the most positive experience in coming to the pain clinic?
We have taken John a few times and found them understanding

and as helpful as they could be — that is, trying different drugs. From memory, it has been a few years since we have been there but most of the drugs did not help much. Maybe we should try again soon. [Making an appointment as soon as possible would be a good idea, as pain management teams are constantly developing and changing in their use of medications, in particular of opioids, for pain relief.]

What would you like to learn to help you through these hard times?
How to help John with his chronic pain problems.

What support do you hope to receive when your child leaves in-patient care?
No support at all! Only the home-care services I already have in place and sometimes I ask for the community nurses to come and help with dressings etc when needed, but this is never offered. I always organise all help myself.

Are you confident about giving your child the medication as prescribed by the treating physician?
I am, now that the doctor has explained it to me.

Who would you call first if your child suffered a relapse after returning home?
Normally I will call the paediatrician or the hospital that John has been discharged from. If it is a prolonged problem which we have been treating at home, I will ring our GP or take him to casualty.

When your child's illness is diagnosed as terminal

When a family has a seriously ill or injured child, the whole family suffer emotional pain. Grief counselling for the parents and the whole family should be encouraged as soon as the diagnosis is made, so that it is possible to live with her condition, maximising her quality of life each day.

Grief counsellors are specially trained to deal with particular problems. You may have a very good counsellor attached to your hospital facility who will nurture the whole family through this very difficult period. Leora Kuttner's book *A Child in Pain* is one of the definitive books on the subject. Ask the counsellor for a list of further reading.

Ask for help

When your child is suffering from chronic pain and/or is hospitalised, your family and friends will probably phone and ask after him, and might say, 'I wish there was something I could do to help.' You will most likely know if they mean it or not, and if they are in a position to offer help. Don't expect people to read your mind. Why not just jump in and delegate? People may not know what to say or do to help and will really welcome being told what is needed.

It's important that you choose the people around you carefully when you are involved in hospital meetings or supporting the child through painful procedures at home or in hospital. You need to concentrate your time and energy on being with the sick child and taking special care of your other children, who will be finding the situation difficult to deal with. This is where good friends in your network will prove invaluable. Avoid contact with negative people whose opinions may depress you and destroy your confidence.

It is a time when you must work on finding a balance within your own life. The body has its own natural opioids, the endorphins that help you through painful and difficult times. You can release them by smiling, laughter, gentle exercise and spending time only with positive people.

Helen House and respite care

It was my privilege to spend time with the Pickering family, whose beautiful son Harry died at the age of six, and to learn much about Helen House and the assistance it gave them during their most troubled times.

Harry's mother Lizzie had noticed that her baby, although very bright intellectually, lacked the movements she would have expected. He did not begin to crawl and his legs didn't seem to be working properly. She became increasingly anguished that there might be something wrong with the fourteen-month-old after his brother Cameron was born.

Soon after, Harry was diagnosed with spinal muscular atrophy, a neuromuscular disease. The muscular wasting associated with the disease was already evident about a year after the diagnosis. A multi-skilled team, including occupational therapists and nurses, helped his family care for Harry and provided them with support. When faced with such a terrible reality on a day-to-day basis, the practical management of a very ill child — in this case, combined with bringing up another healthy, vigorous child — is extremely difficult for any parent.

This is where Helen House, a respite home for children in Oxford, England, came into its own. Respites and hospices for children differ in many ways from hospices for adults. The illnesses are different, the period of terminal care is often much longer, the number of people affected by the patient's illness is larger and respite care for the whole family is essential.

Harry's family was able to go to the respite every six weeks or so for a long weekend. Helen House is like a comfortable family home with brightly decorated rooms. The sick child has his own bedroom and is cared for by the home's staff so his parents and siblings can go to a separate flat and have a break. At home they would never get a full night's rest because Harry required turning over in bed every two hours and constant attention when he was awake, which was not only physically exhausting but also very tough emotionally. Without access to a respite facility, parents can sink into despair or suffer breakdowns. As many as 86 per cent of marriages fail under the strain of caring for a child who has a terminal illness.

When Harry was two and a half, he was enrolled in the local nursery school, which was attached to the primary school he later attended. It was difficult for young and inexperienced teachers to deal with the fact that Harry had a terminal disease and could die at any time. His lungs were very weak and in winter he was prone to frequent bouts of pneumonia. Harry was never able to walk, so right from the beginning he required a sophisticated electric wheelchair. The other children quickly accepted Harry and his wheelchair and never distinguished between him and their other playmates, including him in all the activities.

As his condition worsened, morphine was prescribed to ease the pain of breathing and swallowing. Harry did understand that he would have a limited life, although the word 'death' was not used in his presence until the very last months of his life. He was in excruciating pain and having great difficulty breathing and swallowing. 'Mummy,' he said, a few days before he died, 'I think I would like to be not at home or in hospital, but at Helen House, so would you take me there please?'

Helen House is closely associated with the Radcliffe Infirmary, one of the major hospitals in England, and provides specialist paediatric palliative care and medicines to keep the dying child in as much comfort as possible.

After the death of their child, the family may remain at the respite home until they feel ready to leave. There will be long grieving, and bereavement counselling is a very important part of the service that Helen House offers. The counselling for the parents and siblings continues as and when required for a long period of time.

Douglas House

Douglas House was opened in 2005 when Sister Frances, who started Helen House, recognised the need for children of fourteen and over to be treated in a different environment — as 'guests' rather than patients — and they are cared for there until the age of forty. This is particularly important for sufferers of tumours and multiple sclerosis, as well as motor neurone disease. The adult hospices do not cater specifically for this age group, so the innovative care at Douglas House is very important. A remark from a mother of a patient at Douglas House explains how those at both houses feel about the respices: 'For me, it's a place where I don't have to put on a brave face. I can just let it all go. The staff here know if you're bluffing about how you're really feeling and, before you know it, the barriers that you're so used to keeping up come down.'

Website: http://www.helenanddouglas.org.uk

The BBC has screened an eight-part TV series, 'The Children of Helen and Douglas House'. See http://www.bbc.co.uk/religion/programmes/misc/helenhouse.html

.

10

Caring for Those with Chronic Pain

When you are caring for someone who is ill, it is important to understand the nature of that person's illness and the type of pain and discomfort they are experiencing. It is crucial to have a good relationship with their general practitioner, who can explain the diagnosis and prognosis, the treatment for the symptoms, and coordinate specialist advice. A GP is best positioned to help you make balanced decisions about the future, being aware of your personal and family circumstances, and hopefully is able to provide home visits if needed.

Rather than shying away from obtaining information, seek to learn as much as you can, because what you learn will help you know what to do.

For life-limiting illnesses, there are specific booklets available from your GP or specialist which will give details of many diagnosed illnesses, and these booklets will give the initial information needed. They usually include details of help lines, web addresses and means of contacting respite services.

The challenges

In caring for others, you need to be aware of and respect other people's different ways of dealing with difficulties and challenges as they arise, ways that may have developed with long experience. If a sick person is slow to seek help, encouragement is more useful than scolding. Otherwise you may project your own anxieties on to them, feeding them with your own fears. Serious illness brings out your own personal vulnerabilities.

As stated previously, pacing the day is the secret to making the most of each moment — and that applies as much to the carer as to the person being cared for. Mapping out one day at a time, taking each hour as it comes, works well. But it is also essential to have an overall plan of activities and treatment options that will allow the carer some time for leisure and to pursue work and family business.

You may fear that you will discover something about an illness or disability with which you cannot cope. Ignorance will not protect you from the problems, and knowledge will allow you to make your day as active as you can within realistic limitations. Most sick people want to stay in their own homes as long as is practical, retaining their independence and preferring to be surrounded by familiar belongings and for friends to be free to visit at their convenience. Generally, health authorities facilitate this: from their point of view, it is cheaper to provide ancillary services for domestic and nursing help in the home than it is to take a person into full-time care.

For the carer (as well as the patient), worries about the financial implications of the illness can be particularly stressful. If the carer can no longer participate in activities that are income-producing or relaxing, it can lead to depression. These same problems can lead to anxiety about the future: how will you cope yourself, who will provide for you and for the patient, and will community care be available? All of these are problems that the GP can assist with, and it is important to raise them and get help.

The doctor or home carer team (see below) can also help arrange respite care, which is designed to give the carer a break. It can either be care in a day-centre, support in the home for a few hours a week, or a short stay in a residential respite facility.

Home services

Difficult though this will be, if you are able to it is better to care for patients in their own home. There are many back-up services provided by local councils and a few excellent respite care places.

Your local council or GP can arrange for a home-care assessment team to visit the home and work out if any specialist care or equipment is needed, provide information on suitable care options and help arrange access or referral to appropriate residential or community care if necessary. This usually means an occupational therapist, a physiotherapist and a social worker will visit and see if the furniture is suitable (they may provide an electrically operated armchair to help the patient sit and stand with ease, or a specially designed bed). They will also assess whether aids for getting out of bed, for showering and for mobility are required. In some cases these aids will be provided free of charge, sometimes the patient may have to contribute to their cost. If you are going to require a team of day carers to come and go, allow for the weaknesses of human nature, and keep items of sentimental or financial value safely hidden or locked away.

If the patient has a terminal illness, a palliative care team will usually be assigned to her. The team is ideally placed to coordinate the medical, nursing, physio, dietary and other needs of the person, and it is much better that all of these different matters are being handled in a coordinated way.

Arrangements can be made for the district nurse to call as frequently as twice a day if your patient is at home and unable to handle medication safely. Community aid for shopping and cleaning is usually means tested but check with your health fund if anything can be claimed back (usually there is a set limit per annum, depending on the fund). Some local councils run or help with a shopping service, or this may have to be done by a paid agency. Ask your local shops if they will deliver to the sick: often they will provide this service free of charge for orders over a certain limit; sometimes they charge a set fee.

If you are considering home care, ensure you have respite-care options available (see page 160). You will need to be assessed as a family for this. It provides a back-up should you, as principal carer, fall ill yourself, have another emergency to attend to or simply need a holiday. Most respite homes accept patients for a minimum of one week. Increased funding is being allocated to improve this vital service. Respite is also offered for short time-outs so the carer can have a few hours off. If there are no respite services in your area, campaign for them earnestly. There are also a number of support groups for carers, so they can meet or phone someone to unburden themselves in total confidence; ask your GP for referrals.

Legal issues

It is important that a person with a terminal illness makes a legally binding will — and it is your duty of care to ensure that those you love do this. The will can include details about how the person wishes to be treated at various stages of the illness, or a separate 'living will' can be made that makes it clear whether or not the person wishes to be resuscitated should the need arise. (Ambulance staff and accident and emergency departments may override this request, as it is their duty of care to resuscitate a patient.)

Many people are unhappy at the notion of writing a will, fearing they are being taken advantage of, or that their death is more imminent than it really is. This is quite a normal reaction, but many bereaved families live in financial hardship because this simple step has not been taken.

Physical care

When a person is in pain, it is vitally important that medication is given at the right time, and you must follow the instructions concerning when to take food — before or after, or even with — because absorption differs with various substances. Keep a notebook by the bed in which you can record each dose and the time it was given. This is an efficient way to do things and should work best for patient and carer. Your local pharmacist may be able to organise the dispensation of tablets into special plastic boxes with the days and times marked.

Most people crave independence and so patients must find coping mechanisms, especially if bowel and bladder factors begin to enter into the picture. Specialist nurses are employed and paid for by the health authorities to make home visits to assess incontinence problems and to advise on the best medications and aids to keep you as comfortable as possible.

A carer must be aware of the way stress and embarrassment, especially in public places, can worsen symptoms such as the tremors that are associated with Parkinson's disease. An important decision a carer needs to make is whether to do the shopping for someone whose movements are limited and who can only move very slowly, or whether to spend much more time actually accompanying the person shopping. Discussing this with the person helps: he may have a preference. But be aware that he may just not want to be a trouble to you, or may be ashamed to be seen in public with his limitations (which may be compounded if he has incontinence problems and is afraid of venturing out of the house for fear of 'having an accident'). Don't be afraid to be a little assertive in the face of this reticence. Embarrassment and shame can be overcome if the person is encouraged to get used to being out and about. Staying at home may encourage him to turn in on himself (doctors speak of 'involution'), losing interest in the world and becoming depressed.

With some diseases, there may also be swallowing problems. In extreme cases, swallowing is so painful and difficult that the patient must be fed through a gastric tube. The tube will be used for liquefied medicine, as well as for nutritional supplements. Carers must be trained by a nurse or doctor how to fill the gastro-intestinal feed tube and some may see this as something beyond their ability. However, the procedure is relatively simple and can be learned with the hospital treating team at the time the tube is inserted by the gastroenterology department.

Things to consider when seeking a nursing home

You may not be in a position to care for the patient at home. Before you look for an alternative, consult your GP and other medical professionals for advice. Check your local council for details of approved nursing homes. Take your time when choosing a home because this is an important step for you and for the patient.

Inspect several homes. This can be time-consuming, depressing and may even appear to be hopeless. But persist, because it is essential that the best permanent place be found for the patient so that if her condition worsens she will not have to move to another building or facility. Time spent now will avoid further upset and much wasted money. Some government-funded homes are required to retain a number of places for those living on a low income. If your patient is in this category, check exactly what will be covered by the low fee she will pay (possibly pension only). You may have to pay an additional fee to employ a dedicated night nurse from an agency.

Find out about medical services. Make sure your chosen medical providers are welcome at the home. Good nursing homes will have close relationships with a number of health professionals. You need to know what health services are provided and that those providing them are qualified.

Enquire about staffing levels. Be cautious about reports written to impress visiting inspectors. By prior agreement, they always appear at an appointed time, so staff levels may be artificially increased for the inspectors' visits.

Speak to the staff. Weigh up in your own mind how involved they are with those in their care. This way you will also be able to evaluate any signs of racism or discrimination against certain groups of patients, particularly those in the lower income group.

Speak to other families whose patients are in the home. Ask them how things are going. This will give you an idea of how your patient will be treated.

Look around the premises. Check out the kitchen and ask to see a typical week's menus. Often the main meal is in the middle of the day with a light evening meal served as early as 4.30 p.m. Ask if there is a chance of the patient being given a snack during the night if it's needed. Your patient may be unable to feed without help: find out if there is staff to do this.

Emotional care

Sexuality

Just because a person is in pain does not mean his sexual desire leaves him. There is a role here for specialised understanding. Some patients may gain great satisfaction simply from hugging. Touching remains an important instinctive part of being human.

To deny sick people that loving touch is to deny them a very healing force.

Guilt

When interviewing patients, I have found that, young and old, they all complained of one prevalent emotion: guilt. Children as young as four said they felt guilty because they had leukaemia — they felt it was a punishment for something they had done wrong. Patients who were terminally ill felt guilty about being burdensome to their carer or partner.

The carer/partners also felt guilty about being inadequate, guilty whenever they felt angry about losing their independence, and guilty whenever they left the patient in the care of someone else or, through sheer exhaustion, had to take them to respite care for a week or two.

Fear and confusion

The person in pain may be confused by the changing state of her illness, not knowing what to expect and how the illness is progressing. Another emotion shared by both carer and sufferer is fear. Both feel fearful of the present and of the future. How will they cope with the pain, with the bereavement? What will happen if or when the condition worsens? How will they face death?

By sharing your experiences and contacting other people with the disease and their carers, you can gain strength and confidence and begin new friendships. Or you may wish to speak with a counsellor who really understands the disease.

The role of the advocate

With many diseases, the patient ideally requires an advocate, who may be a friend or relative, to speak for him. This is because medical staff are overburdened with many seriously ill patients, requiring lengthy periods of one-on-one care. Often, even in the best of hospices and nursing homes, it may be up to half an hour before a nurse can attend to the needs of a very ill patient, because of something as simple as remaking the bed of an incontinent patient or being involved in a team medical evaluation. Due to chronic understaffing in most hospitals, this is inevitable. More money needs to be allocated to this vital service and more hospices are required for people of all ages. And more nurses who have empathy with geriatric patients should be recruited.

Jeremy has a group of friends who have visited regularly for eighteen months. He has suffered moments of panic when no nurse was able to answer his call, particularly through the night when terrifying nightmares overcame him. So he asked for a friend or relative to stay the night. Often it is possible to put a camp bed in the patient's room or at least an easy chair in which the friend can doze while keeping company and being on call to help. Someone to read to you, to hold your hand, to mop your brow during moments of terror makes a great difference in offering comfort and reassurance.

In many countries, it is the norm to have a relative or friend present to assist with washing and feeding and non-nursing duties. Having a loved one present comforts the patient, easing anxiety. However, it can be difficult for friends to be available for this loving work of care. If family members are to take periods of leave from work to do this, in my opinion, at least they should be entitled to the meagre carers' benefit, which should not be means tested as it is at present.

One solution is to organise a group of friends who will follow a roster and even bring tasty meals in occasionally to offer relief from institutional hospital food. About sixteen people are needed if the patient is in for a long stay. That way each person only has to do a meal and a visit once a fortnight, and there are two 'spare' friends to call on if the roster gets out of kilter. It is an enriching experience to be an advocate for a patient at the end of her life.

If a group of people are involved in care-giving, one person should be chosen as the official spokesperson for the patient, otherwise it is confusing for medical staff. In any case, all advocacy should be conducted with politeness and calm, because, reasonably, the medical staff will not take kindly to being told 'how to treat' the patient. But the advocate does have to speak up on behalf of the patient if something is obviously going wrong. For example, if the person you are caring for vomits all her oral medication, the nursing staff may have to await the doctors' rounds before they are permitted to introduce breakthrough pain relief. Obviously, stabilising the patient's severe pain is essential to reduce needless suffering — this should be raised with the palliative care team and a workable solution found.

A woman who was advocate for her aged mother reported that 'I was totally happy with Mum's care except that in the last few days, when a crisis occurred, there was always a time lag in her receiving breakthrough pain relief "until a doctor called to write it up". At one stage, when Mum was almost comatose, she was actually baring her teeth like a tiger in pain before adequate relief was given to her.' She suggests that 'places such as nursing homes and rehabilitation units which do not have a resident doctor should always have scripts pre-written for breakthrough pain relief. Crises always occur at unexpected and inconvenient times, and these need to be anticipated and prepared for.'

If a group of friends is providing support, it is a good idea to keep a notebook by the patient's bedside so whoever attends can record important details and problems, which can then be seen by attending medical staff and visitors and acted upon if need be. (Include a drug routine chart in the notebook. This should be followed scrupulously and if on your shift you note the medical staff have been unable to give an injection or tablet at the prescribed time or have not signed it up in their book, you are entitled to point this out and ensure the patient receives medication on time — but check by asking in a way not to offend.) It is a way of keeping the group in touch with progress or deterioration. Any change in circumstances must be reported immediately to the nursing unit manager or, if the patient is home-based and has a terminal illness, to the assigned palliative care team.

Peter and MS

Multiple sclerosis (often called MS) affects how the brain and spinal cord send and receive messages to and from other parts of the body. Many of the nerve fibres in the body are covered by a 'myelin sheath' (think of the insulation around an electrical wire to give you an idea) that allows these messages to travel more quickly along the nerve. In multiple sclerosis, these myelin sheaths are progressively, though unpredictably, destroyed.

This can lead to loss of function of muscles, in the legs, arms and fingers, even the muscles that control actions such as swallowing, the tongue movement that allows speech, and eye muscles and eyelids. It may start as weakness of the affected areas, and go on to complete paralysis in the most severe cases. Muscle spasms are common. Nerves carrying sensations to the brain can also be affected, leading to the loss of vision, to facial pain, to widespread electric shock or tingling sensations, or to loss of sensation.

The disease can appear to get better ('remit') and then get worse again ('relapse'). For many, major symptoms do not present for years or ever, and the only sign of the disease is a slight limp or slowing of pace. However, often it is inexorably progressive, with loss of control of body functions, including of the bladder and bowel.

Because of altered sensation, neuralgia and muscle spasm, some patients may suffer considerable pain. But for many others, it is facing the reality of their situation that can be the most challenging. To make matters worse, in cases where the patient is unable to speak, it is very difficult to assess the exact needs and to get 'ahead of the pain'. Reaction to drugs that may adversely affect the patient must be monitored by a specialist in MS care, so routine visits to a neurologist are essential — ideally home visits, as moving the patient can often cause the pain to increase greatly. Few nursing homes set up for geriatric care have these facilities, so for the younger MS patient such as Peter, who was in the nursing home from the ages of thirty-eight to forty-one, life was one long series of painful experiences, helped mainly by the dedicated and devoted care of immediate family members.

For carers of those with MS, the deterioration of the patient is devastating and the emotional pain involved in observing that breakdown is considerable, not to mention the extreme physical pressures of 24-hour care.

Fiona, along with her mother, has provided care for her brother Peter. She explains what being a carer involves.

Fiona describes looking after her brother

What carers need to provide — unerringly and unhesitatingly: Love and loving care with unending hope and positive attitude: this can be hard when faced with possible incapacitation and loss of dignity in worst-case scenarios.

Humour — often. How things are handled can be a magical element to a sufferer's level of coping. A laugh and a giggle can be very therapeutic and a great distraction. It can also alleviate symptoms on some levels.

Dignity can be lost or threatened in such a debilitating condition. With organs possibly failing at some stage, depending on the type and stage of MS (relapsing remitting, non-relapsing remitting, primary progressive, secondary progressive), the basic human abilities such as going to the toilet can be threatened. If a carer can provide assistance in a practical, caring manner, a sufferer's dignity can be maintained.

The importance of information: The cause of MS is unknown but can begin as early as early teens although the effects or symptoms may not show until much later such as mid-thirties or forties.

As a family of carers, we found the more we knew the more we could help. With correct diagnosis (which is through eradicating most if not all other alternatives), we set to work on planning how we could help. We searched the internet almost on a daily basis for new information and had alerts set up from the MS Society websites to let us know when new research or developments came to light.

Lack or reduction of stress: Mental and physical stress exacerbates MS symptoms. If carers can try to lessen emotional, mental and physical stress they can at least help reduce its effects on the sufferer. Any anguish experienced can produce disastrous results such as catatonic states in severe cases.

Stimulation: As I understand it, research has shown that keeping the brain active and functioning can delay or slow the process of MS. Chess, crosswords, quiz games could be played and general knowledge exercised by reading (or being read) the newspaper to keep abreast of news. This reassures the sufferer that he can still function on every level for as long as possible. Stimulation in audio and visual ways can be provided to complement other forms of stimulation such as humour and general loving, caring support and company. Audio tapes of music and/or books can provide company if 24-hour assistance or company is not possible. (Public libraries usually have a stock of books on tape or CD.)

Complementary therapies: Acupuncture (consistent and continuous), regular deep tissue and relaxation massage, physiotherapy and reflexology can all make a difference as can a good Chinese medical practitioner. With MS, circulation can be affected at any stage, and acupuncture and herbal remedies can assist effectively. Check with the neurologist before administering any herbal remedies, though, as they may not interact well with prescribed medication. TENS machines that deliver low-level electrical pulses to damaged nerves can be very effective as they interrupt pain messages caused by damaged nerves.

Physical exercise: Mental and physical stimulation can be complemented by gentle physical exercise. This must be measured by quantity and level of difficulty. A sufferer should maintain flexibility and movement where possible. Walking and swimming are best but at any point that the person feels physically stressed (gets out of breath or starts sweating, for instance), it is vital to reduce the exertion. Any extremes of temperature can lead to symptom increase.

Mobility can be the key to ensuring independence for a person suffering from any disabling disease. The use of walking sticks (prior to wheelchairs, if required) can allow greater flexibility and lessen reliance on another person. One of the greatest challenges for MS sufferers is the decline in mobility and increase in reliance upon carers. It can be so important to try to ensure that people can still walk to the shops, or have access to transport that lets them do 'the basics' like going for a coffee, or out for a drink or dinner, doing the shopping. Although carers can do their best to support people going through most of these phases, it is also important to support their wishes to be as independent as is practically possible. But denial of their disease or symptoms is common. Installation of such things as ramps or support rails can allow greater independence, but sometimes can confirm not only the presence of the disease but the effects of it on their everyday lives. Anything in its extreme — mentally, emotionally, physically — can lead to an episode worsening. One of the added strains on the sufferer and carers is the total unpredictability of the stages of deterioration.

Food and liquids: Assisting in the diet of sufferers can be a vital element of a carer's role. MS symptoms can be limited to some extent by reducing lactose and/or gluten intake and sometimes dairy products. Sufferers must never dehydrate or overheat or suffer from the cold, as these states can be disastrous, aggravating symptoms and even sometimes ending in hospitalisation. Even a hot bath can do this, although the aggravation is usually only temporary. They need plenty of fresh fruit juices, water, indeed any liquid excluding alcohol and caffeine. Limited alcohol can be acceptable as a very occasional treat but, again, exacerbates symptoms very easily.

Rest: A sufferer must listen to his body and rest regularly. As mentioned, excesses of any kind of stress can worsen symptoms. An afternoon nap is suggested, with early bedtimes (although insomnia can be a problem — but if this is the case your GP or neurologist can prescribe sleeping tablets to help). It has been found useful to provide eye patches and ear plugs as well.

Depression: With diagnosis of any debilitating disease, depression can be a factor. Carers must be aware of signs and act quickly. Hopefully sufferers have a circle of loving family and friends around them to care for and support them, but sometimes this is not always the case.

Company: A great way to provide care twenty-four hours

a day without exhaustion on the carer's side can be to organise a rota of visitors (but not too many). People are more than happy to help for an hour or so once a week.

Peter's mother talks about MS

Pain increases as muscles fail to receive messages from the brain and become less and less able to stimulate movement, as the myelin sheathes become scarred. This may cause pain that could range from manageable to extreme. Bowel and bladder function, speech, swallowing and memory function may all be affected.

Diet: We give him Vitamin B12 and other supplements. Mealtimes are important, so make sure food is tasty and attractive.

Memory: It helps to have a whiteboard, or similar, with clearly indicated daily events, for activities, comings and goings, names of carers and times. This avoids confusion and anxiety. It must be large enough with clear lettering for the patient, whose eyesight may be failing, to read without difficulty, and it should be placed in a position easily viewed from the bed or wheelchair.

Diary: Record pain levels, any changes, concerns or anxieties as it is often hard to recall retrospectively.

Energy: Conserve and use in a planned way.

Intimate care: Peter found that roles needed to be clearly demarcated between wife and mother and carers. He did not like us to be responsible for toileting or catheter changes. Others may feel differently, but I guess it comes down to maintaining dignity.

Key words: Love, dignity, self-esteem, humour, care, inclusion, stimulation, information, knowledge, respect, empathy, communication, company. And of these, the most vital is love.

Talk: Because the MS sufferer may become more limited in speech, memory, movement, and so on, it remains vital to communicate. He/she must remain part of everyday life and you, the carer, are the pathway. Even those unable to speak may be allowed to communicate through love, humour, respect and the giving of dignity. Being included in conversations with those in the room, even if the patient cannot communicate by speech, can be done by a loving touch to the arm or shoulder, and eye contact must be made too — something many visitors are uncomfortable with — to involve the patient, who has an opportunity to react by blinking, nodding or by whatever means she/he is able to show involvement.

Fight for your loved one by developing awareness of the latest in research and treatment. This may be easier for you, as carer, to do than the MS sufferers. Their sense of emotional well-being may be enhanced when there is understanding from the people who love them, when they know, or instinctively feel, that no stone is being left unturned. This gives hope and confidence.

11

When Pain Becomes
a Battleground

Two important problems well illustrate just how pain itself can become a battleground. In repetitive strain injuries (RSI; also known as occupational overuse injuries or OOS) the pain is the main symptom; in myalgic encephalomyelitis, also known as chronic fatigue syndrome (ME/CFS), pain is one important symptom among many.

In each case, the illness has been given different names at different times and in different places. Exactly how they are caused is in dispute or simply unknown, but there is no doubt the symptoms represent something real. And at various times, members of the medical profession, the media or the courts have expressed doubts about the sufferings of people with these two problems, portraying them as psychologically disturbed or even malingerers.

Even when they are strong enough to stand up to their critics, people with unexplained pain symptoms are forced into a 'siege mentality' and much of their energy is spent defending themselves against scepticism and disbelief. Of course, this does great harm to their prospects of recovery. Others may feel guilty and, as Dr Henri Rubenstein argues, 'Guilt destroys the defences. A guilty patient is often unable to find enough energy to defend his body.'

I know all about this because I suffer from a disorder called adhesive arachnoiditis, which has no outward signs but causes severe, chronic and intractable pain. It is caused by the inflammation of one of the spinal cord coverings (meninges), the middle meninges, the arachnoid and nerve roots. This inflammation causes the covering to become 'sticky', so it adheres to the spinal cord and the nerve roots as they exit the spinal canal, which in turn stick to the meninges — source of the pain. Adhesive arachnoiditis can be progressive in some cases. It can also cause loss of motor function, numbness, tingling, loss of bladder and bowel function, the sensation of walking on rocks or glass, burning, groin pain and can, in some rare instances, cause paralysis. There is currently no cure for adhesive arachnoiditis, and no treatment other than pain management. And living with the disorder involves constantly arming yourself against the disbelievers.

ME/CFS: 'The disease of a thousand names'

As well as enduring severe, unexplained fatigue, people suffering from ME/CFS often have chronic pain. They experience all the frustrations and difficulties of having insufficient 'proof' for a concrete diagnosis and therefore of not always being believed, which is so insulting and frightening. Interestingly, sufferers say they are afraid to admit to having ME/CFS lest it ruin their employment chances.

You cannot diagnose an illness when it has no name. Yet once it is given a name, suddenly it is found everywhere. In the mid-1980s there was an explosion in cases of chronic fatigue syndrome (CFS), raising fears that there was an epidemic of a new illness. Some suggested it was mass hysteria and, because it often struck young people after a viral illness, it was given the uncharitable name 'yuppie 'flu'. There were fears this was some new virus, some new environmental toxin.

But it wasn't new. The English sweats, post-polio syndrome, neurasthenia, Raggedy Anne syndrome, Akureyri disease, Royal Free disease (after the London hospital), La Spasmophilie, Tapanui 'flu (after the New Zealand town), chronic fatigue syndrome and a host of other names have been used at different times for what is probably the same condition. Many of these names were invented after reported epidemics (more than fifty documented since 1934). Currently, the Americans insist on the name chronic fatigue syndrome. The English call it myalgic encephalomyelitis (literally, inflammation of the brain and spinal cord leading to muscular aches and pains). A compromise is to call it ME/CFS.

It is not classified as a disease because its causes and mechanisms — its 'pathology' — have not been worked out. It might be called a syndrome, a cluster of symptoms and signs with a certain pattern in time ('syndrome' is often used in medicine as an explanation when details seem rather vague).

What is ME/CFS?

The experts are still arguing about the definition of ME/CFS, but it has a number of characteristic 'flu-like symptoms: aches and pains, ranging from joint and muscular aches and pains to head-aches, sore throat and enlarged lymph nodes; 'brain fog'— difficulty concentrating and with memory, so-called 'cognitive dysfunction'; being unable to tolerate lights and sounds (so-called 'sensory storms') — known as photosensitivity; disturbed sleep; fatigue, worsened by exercise and exertion; and it often follows a viral ill-ness, especially in young people.

Some experts believe one of the big problems that is causing unnecessary confusion is concentration on unexplained fatigue as the main symptom of ME/CFS. Everyone has fatigue from time to time, when sick, run-down, depressed, short on sleep or over-worked. And many serious illnesses cause fatigue. If fatigue is used as the starting point in diagnosing this illness, all the known causes of fatigue have to be eliminated first. Then only the unexplained causes are left. As one sceptic said: first you have to exclude all those who show any real 'hard' evidence of disease before you can diagnose ME/CFS. So ME/CFS ends up being a general term, full of left-over cases often with no hard evidence of disease.

Doctors may be unfamiliar with much of the research in the field, and may take a simplistic and unsympathetic view of this 'new' illness. ME/CFS is frustrating for physicians too, requiring them to spend a lot of time and to give much emotional support. It is easier to conclude that what cannot be properly explained is a psychological problem.

Pain and ME/CFS

Pain is a major part of ME/CFS, and there is probably a degree of overlap with other causes of chronic pain causing fatigue. And fatigue and sleep disturbance can worsen pain, making it harder to cope with. It should be no surprise that these form a kind of vicious cycle.

Commonly described types of pain in ME/CFS are: a 'flu-like feeling, with aching muscles and joints; various bladder and pelvic pains, particularly in women; nagging neck and chest pains; feelings like ants in the skin; various stabbing pains; pains experienced in joints and bones (although these might be 'referred' from somewhere else); pain and problems such as constipation associated with irritable bowel syndrome; fibromyalgic pain involving aches, sometimes sickening in intensity, in the muscles particularly when they are pressed; and various forms of headaches, including pains behind the eyes, in the ears, hypersensitivity of the teeth and pains in the jaw.

Causes of ME/CFS

It is believed that some people with ME/CFS have been exposed to certain virus or bacteria (such as rickettsia, in some parts of the world); others might also have been exposed to various chemicals or toxins or been vaccinated with a poorly tested vaccine (like the 'Gulf War syndrome' cases of veterans from the 1991 war, who were deloused and vaccinated thoroughly, although their illness might be related to possible exposure to germs common in the Middle East region). Some sufferers may be chronically infected with viruses that cannot be routinely detected. Some but not all have experienced major stress before or during exposure to an infection or possible toxin. Many, possibly most, suffer from food or chemical sensitivities. A minority experience major depression.

Some researchers note changes in muscle function in the people they study; others find ME/CFS sufferers have no such changes. Some people have signs of ongoing activity in their immune systems. Some have subtle hormone (like thyroid problems) or blood pressure changes, and some don't. Researchers have found changes in heart function, muscle function, the blood cells and in the function of the stomach and intestines — but not always in all people, and often using tests that are not widely available.

There are few practicable treatments for these 'changes' and, if there are, the treatments either haven't been researched fully or get indifferent results.

Different ways of looking at ME/CFS

Some researchers think it would be easier to understand the disease if the problems in the central nervous system were taken as the starting point for ME/CFS, rather than fatigue, which is part of so many other diseases and illnesses. It would also remove some of the stigma attached to people who are described as 'chronically fatigued'.

It has been suggested that ME/CFS be renamed Florence Nightingale disease. After her work in the Crimea, Nightingale suffered a chronic ME/CFS-type illness, which may have been a virus or some other illness like typhus, for most of the rest of her life. Attaching her name to the disease could help counterbalance its negative image and also be a reminder that it has been around for a long time.

Another approach is to stop searching for a single cause and a single treatment. ME/CFS is probably a complex reaction of the body's immune and nervous systems to any of a number of different stressors, or combinations of stressors (which might include toxins, infections, vaccines, psychological stress). One model attempts to pull this all together by thinking of ME/CFS as the body's normal defensive response to a variety of 'attacks' — by germs and/or toxins and/or stress — involving a whole cascade of subtle chemical changes that put the body in chronic defence mode in a way that is exhausting and unhelpful.

Types of treatments on offer

The principles are the same as for all chronic pain.

If you have ME/CFS, you may become depressed with your situation and the limitations on your lives. Antidepressants may help if there is depression, but do not benefit everyone; indeed, you may be highly sensitive to the effects of medicines such as antidepressants. Antidepressants may also help with sleep and pain for those with ME/CFS who have no depression: this is similar to the situation with chronic pain of other types.

The majority of doctors now agree that ME/CFS is not caused by depression — and that depression is more likely to be an effect of the illness.

Some people with ME/CFS have gained some benefit from 'graded exercise' programs, in which the participants start with a few minutes exercise and over the course of months work up to, say, thirty minutes per day. However, most studies have been done on people who were well enough to participate in the treatment: people with more severe illness may not benefit and, indeed, it might well make them worse.

As with all chronic pain, people may be so desperate that they will be tempted to try a variety of unproven remedies. Interestingly there are quite a few doctors who specialise in ME/CFS who also try some unproven treatments. These include: colonic irrigation; long courses of antibiotics; medicines to alter blood pressure, thyroid and other hormones; anti-candida diets; possibly excessive amounts of vitamins and mineral supplements, and amino-acid supplements. Often there is a reasonable sounding theory behind the treatment and sometimes the patients report benefits, but unless proper studies are done it is impossible to know.

The ME/CFS battleground

In the nineteenth century, doctors were comfortable using the terms 'neurasthenia' or 'exhaustion of the nerve cells': this was thought to be a real physical problem with the nerves. People with what we now call ME/CFS would probably have received this diagnosis. Many a Victorian novel (and household) had a mysterious bed-ridden invalid upstairs, who might be spied prowling around when everyone else had gone to bed. A modern reader might tend to think she (it was almost always a 'she') was malingering. A person suffering ME/CFS would understand better: late at night may be the time when he finally has a few good hours, made bearable by the darkness and quiet.

Freud made 'weak nerves' unfashionable, and neurasthenia became a psychiatric diagnosis. However, as more information becomes available about disturbances in nerve function in a whole range of illnesses, the pendulum may swing back to the point of view that 'exhaustion of the nerve cells' has a physiological basis.

It wouldn't be the first time that medical advances have found an organic basis for what was thought to be a psychological problem.

The battle about ME/CFS is in a way about who 'owns' it, a battleground between physicians and psychiatrists with patients caught in the middle, between mainstream health professionals and 'alternative' practitioners. The best advice is to leave the battleground to the doctors as much as possible. Don't be drawn into it.

RSI, compensation and pain

Insurance companies have often assumed that claimants exaggerate pain 'for financial gain'. One of the most disputed injuries is repetitive strain injury (RSI), also known as occupational overuse injury (OOS), which is commonly associated with the workplace. Over the years, sufferers have been given many derogative names and the condition is still regarded as controversial. But it is a very real and painful injury sustained by many.

This is not a new condition but a symptom or group of symptoms from which humankind has suffered over the ages. The great composer Robert Schumann suffered an overuse injury from a device intended to strengthen his fourth finger which caused such damage that he could no longer pursue a career as a concert pianist due to pain. Michelangelo suffered years of excruciating back and neck pain because of his work on the Sistine Chapel. The nineteenth-century novelists vividly described working conditions that gave rise to repetitive strain injuries. The weavers and millers, the farm threshers, the sheep shearers over-used muscles and tendons as they toiled to earn a living.

All over the world people still engage in manual tasks in fields and factories, building roads and digging holes. Dentists and violinists suffer severe nerve compression following years of occupational strain. We inflict such injuries upon ourselves by using our computers without setting them up suitably. Office workers sitting in front of computers may suffer from RSI in the arms, back and neck unless they are properly advised and take direction seriously.

During our lifetime, many of us will suffer from symptoms of RSI. It is important to recognise the degree of severity at the onset of symptoms and to consult a doctor as soon as you experience aching, tenderness, swelling, pain, tingling or numbness in the arms, neck, fingers or back. Optimistically, it is possible that simple adjustments to work practices may completely solve the problem before the condition becomes serious.

RSI is a general rather than a specific diagnosis and includes many specific injuries, among which are carpal tunnel syndrome, tenosynovitis, tendonitis and nerve entrapment. Medical treatment may include sessions of physiotherapy, injections with steroids, and the prescription of painkillers and/or anti-inflammatory drugs. In extreme cases surgery may be required.

In Australia many years ago, some employers used to refer to those with hand injuries as 'kangaroo paws', of which there was a high incidence. Whether this was due to a high incidence of long shift hours being worked on machinery in overheated work stations, or whether it was simply bad luck, is a matter of anecdote rather than empirical study. Nowadays, workplaces are covered by occupational health and safety acts that oblige employers to provide safe working conditions. But managements will differ in their attitudes to cost and injury, and many people still suffer repetitive strain injuries at work because of bad work practices and unsatisfactory equipment.

Compensation does offer small comfort to those with irreparable industrial injuries, but it is far more cost effective for management to install satisfactory work practices and to prevent RSI in the first instance.

Job rotation is useful (and helps create a multi-skilled workplace), but is rarely practicable. Attention to posture and seating is of prime importance. Ergonomically designed furniture that can be adjusted to different heights is helpful, and simple steps can often be taken to adjust the height of a monitor or the slant of a machine. Inexpensive wrist pads, back rolls and work stands can help avoid hand and neck strains.

Managements differ in their attitudes to injuries and workplace safety. The more enlightened understand upholding their legal obligations, including having a duty of care to employees, is cost-effective. For instance, where a worker suffers an asthma attack that can be directly attributed to working in a smoke-filled environment, the employer can be responsible for medical fees and compensation; therefore, it is in his interest that staff work in a smoke-free environment. Likewise, an employee required to work at a poorly designed desk on ill-adjusted computers may develop repetitive strain injuries that could be avoidable.

Responsibility for preventing RSI also lies with each individual (although few workers have the option to choose their equipment or their working hours). For those who spend long periods at keyboards or at machinery, the simplest aid to avoiding RSI is to stand up straight just for a second or two every twenty minutes: the very act of stretching alters the position of the muscles. Once you have developed this regular habit, you will be surprised how your elbows, wrists and shoulders benefit, as does your back and neck. When sitting at a desk, ensure that your chair allows your knees to be at right angles to the floor with your feet straight in front of you. Your arms should rest comfortably just above the waist at right angles to your body, with your forearms and wrists supported. Do not hunch your shoulders. Take your arms off the keyboard or table and shake them down by your side when pausing between tasks.

It is not only at work that people develop overuse injuries. Keen gardeners, tennis players, gymnasts and walkers also suffer from muscle and tendon injuries. Awareness is the key to avoiding repetitive strain, varying your activities at work, home and at play and never ignoring pain, for it is your warning that something is not right.

Taking responsibility for yourself also means avoiding carrying loads in excess of one-tenth of your body weight. Parents will laugh at this, but you should know that when lifting a child, he will 'give' with you and jump a little, whereas an inanimate object of the same weight will be more unmanageable and potentially more injurious to the back. When packing shopping at the supermarket, divide your loads into bags weighing only five kilograms each. You will soon get used to the quantity and your back will love you forever.

Obviously if you suffer from the symptoms of repetitive strain injuries — tingling in the fingers, numbness in limbs, sharp pain or burning sensations — it is essential that you seek medical advice and treatment. You will feel much better about the prognosis if you realise you can do something active about the way you work, which may prevent repetitive injury from occurring again.

One model workplace solution

Twenty years ago, when I worked as health and safety officer for an enlightened management of a television station, we commissioned a study which proved that preventive care for staff with musculature problems was more cost-effective than paying for post-injury treatment.

Several members of the news crew developed painful shoulder injuries from hauling their heavy Betacam video camcorders around in a war zone. A physiotherapist devised muscle-strengthening exercises for them and their work agreements were amended to provide two-hour swimming sessions twice weekly on full pay during the short periods they spent on home territory. The swimming proved beneficial not only for existing injuries but in preventing future problems. It was a simple solution to a painful problem: building up muscles equal to everyday tasks.

Other measures offered to the staff of five hundred included twice-weekly lunch-time exercise classes, and yoga and tai chi. Although fewer than 20 per cent chose to attend classes, many of the staff began going for walks at lunch time. A physiotherapist came twice a year to check ergonomic work stations. Advice was given on posture and the treatment of injury, those requiring assistance could seek help directly at any time, and the cost of care was met by the organisation. An optometrist came yearly to advise on eye strain prevention and the company paid for eye examinations, although individuals were responsible for the cost of prescribed glasses. Lectures were given on various relaxation and exercise techniques such as Alexander and Feldenkrais. The staff was encouraged to seek help and advice when appropriate.

Time lost for treatment of injuries fell dramatically, as did sick leave. For such ideas to succeed, there must be no obligation or favouritism. People can only benefit if they want to be part of the experiment, otherwise they may feel they are being manipulated.

12

The Politics of Pain

There is a widespread fear of opioids. Governments reluctantly allow the legal medical prescribing of morphine and its derivates to alleviate acute and subsequent chronic pain. But there seems to be a fear of causing addiction — or of being sued (or voted out of office) for causing it — that exceeds the responsibility of assisting patients with managing their pain.

The medical profession is not immune from the same fear. As Anne-Marie Vidal points out in her 2002 article 'The Politics of Pain: the controversy surrounding chronic pain and opioids': 'Anyone who lives with chronic pain is acutely aware of many physicians' difficulty in coming to terms with prescribing adequate pain medication.'

Hundreds of thousands of patients worldwide rely on some form of opioids to control pain. Paracetamol is the drug of preference as first-line treatment, considered to be 'less noxious'. Yet in recent years in Britain the sale of paracetamol products has been restricted to quantities of twenty tablets only, the rationale being the aim of preventing suicides among the teenage group.

Although most people probably agree the prescription of potentially addictive substances (Class A, or Schedule 8, depending on the jurisdiction) ought be controlled, there is a good deal of hypocrisy about how some substances are defined as 'drugs' and others are not. It is interesting to stop and take a good look at the inconsistency of some of our laws. Tobacco is highly addictive and dangerous, but it is produced by powerful business interests. Likewise, alcohol causes far more health problems than opioids, yet drinking is almost a test of true national belonging (and a punishable offense in some Muslim countries).

Not so long ago tea was considered to be a strong stimulant (and locked away safe from the servant girls — although that was partly due to its price), and now it is widely regarded as a benign substance. The reverse is true of opioids, which were available virtually over the counter until the early part of the twentieth century. Pressure from the temperance movement and other anti-drug activists in the USA led to the Harrison Narcotics Act of 1914, and gradually opioids became heavily controlled substances in most jurisdictions of the world. It has been argued that this American legislation on narcotics was really aimed against the British, who dominated the opium trade then, and designed as a repressive measure against Hispanics, who used cocaine widely. In Australia and New Zealand, early opium control rhetoric was infused with anti-Chinese sentiments.

Currently cannabis, in nasal spray and tablet forms, is being widely trialled in Europe and Britain to ease the pain of multiple sclerosis. In 1999 I was advised by senior physicians at a university hospital to trial it myself, but at that time it was only available in the weed form and, as I dislike smoking, the notion did not appeal.

There still exist strong moral and political objections to the use of cannabis even for medical reasons, which seems more to do with a fear of hippies than a rational assessment of the benefits and harms of the substance. Cannabis is a drug — but alcohol isn't. What sense is that? People with a moral mission and political agendas cannot keep their hands out of what should be medical business.

Whereas it is probably reasonable that opioid medication be controlled by legislation and medical prescription, there should always be room for individual assessment of the needs of known responsible patients. This sometimes does not happen.

Opiates and opiophobia

People are steeped in prejudice against morphine and opiates. One of my mentors, who is a chronic pain sufferer with multiple tumours, was shunned by some of his formerly close friends when he and his wife mentioned at a private dinner that he was now suffering so much that the doctors had prescribed regular doses of slow-release morphine. Suddenly this dear man, who they had so revered and looked up to for support and comfort in their own troubles, was 'taking drugs'. No amount of rational discussion was going to deprive this judgemental group of their prejudice. Taking drugs was a sin. 'I am shocked,' said one young woman, 'that a man with your knowledge and experience, both as a paramedic and a minister, should fall prey to drug taking.'

It is all in the language. If you consider your friends to be ill-prepared for exact information, it helps to exchange the word 'medication' (or 'medicine') for 'drug' and not be too ready to specify which medicine you are taking — unless you are prepared for a lecture and possibly even rejection. But perhaps it is important to speak out about it, both to teach others and to learn to whom you can turn as true and valued friends.

During one nationwide broadcast recently, I mentioned to the presenter that the only way I got through each day was with my regular dose of morphine. The presenter looked at me in much the way one would had I said 'I have been known to sniff cocaine.' Hoping it would be clear to the audience, I explained carefully that, when prescribed by a doctor for the treatment of pain, opioid medication was appropriate and necessary for the quality of life for thousands of people who, as a result, are able to function reasonably well in work and to live with less pain. But I was cut off abruptly and the presenter changed the subject.

If you or your children require opioids for the treatment of severe and/or chronic pain, it is vitally important that you understand why they are prescribed and that you feel comfortable about taking this medication. The wider the understanding of pain relief, the more educated we shall all be.

Unfortunately morphine is associated with dealers, street corners, dark alleys and 'injecting in toilets'. So it's an easy leap of imagination from an activity that is criminal to, worse still, a patient who is bound to become an addict.

In Britain, once a patient suffering chronic pain has been prescribed opioids, usually in hospital by a specialist or in a pain clinic and occasionally by a GP, it is permissible for telephone repeats to be given for up to six months, at which time the patient must be re-assessed. In France, opioids are controlled more stringently in that it is mandatory for the GP to physically examine the patient once a week and record his blood pressure. This is required even if the patient must take opioids for the rest of his life. It is time-consuming for the GPs but helps to build up a good relationship, one which will be necessary if symptoms become more severe.

Regulations vary in New Zealand and in the Australian states. For example, in New South Wales, under the Poisons Act, if a patient has been prescribed morphine for intractable non-cancer pain while hospitalised or by a specialist physician in pain management, the prescription may be continued. However, the patient must visit her GP, who holds the sole authority to prescribe, once every thirty days. The doctor must phone an authorisation line and quote the patient's serial number for the Medicare authority for subsidised opioids. If a patient moves to another practice or another area, the authority for her prescription of morphine must be transferred.

When children are prescribed opioids, this can be a problem for many parents. A recent interview with the parents of a country child (who had been in hospital for a couple of months following a motor vehicle accident in which she had suffered life-threatening injuries) revealed that her chronic pain was at last being controlled by very low doses of morphine. Jenny was about to be discharged and because of the pain control was able to return to school. Her parents spoke proudly of how well she was doing. But when asked how they felt about her treatment at the hospital, Jenny's father hesitated and then blurted out, 'These stupid doctors are all very well and, yes, my Jenny is better, but how? She's on morphine, isn't she? They are creating an addict of a ten year old already.' Her mother added, sadly, 'So, we are very disappointed in the treatment.'

It seemed necessary to reassure them that the medical regimen would be lessened as Jenny gained full use of her limbs once more and as the pain no longer dictated doses of opioids. The nursing unit manager was called to reassure them. 'Don't go worrying about addiction problems and overdose,' she said. 'The doctors do measure doses very carefully, according to body size and pain requirements, and will have also written to your GP giving her a full history of graduated reduction of medication when this is appropriate. Pain relief is the right of each and every one of us, young and old.'

The parents looked comforted if not convinced. But this scene brought to mind many similar scenes, regularly played out in hospitals. If opioids are the most successful form of pain relief, and they are prescribed by a specialist who understands pain control, take the specialist's advice, and allow the patient to be relatively pain-free. Achieving a pain-free state is the aim.

One of the most interesting advances in pain management in hospitals is patient-controlled analgesia (known as PCA), which is used especially after major surgery. Instead of the doctor speci-fying doses, the patients are able to top up their own morphine by pressing a little button by the bed (although the doctor does control the quantity prescribed in the PCA). Some may think this is an invitation to abuse but, on the contrary, it has been found that patients who have this kind of control end up using less morphine, on average, than those who are left to request pain relief when they feel the need for it.

Having to wait until your pain is bad enough to ask for pain relief is bad medicine. By the time the pain is that bad, it is harder to treat, and as a result it usually takes longer for the medication to have its effect.

Fear of giving opioids underlies all of this. Many doctors are still trained to fear being fooled by a 'junkie'. And nurses do not receive adequate education in the use of opioids and, particularly in the case of young children, they do not understand that doses are carefully related to weight. They are frightened, particularly when challenged by opioid-fearing parents, even to give the dose recommended by the pain specialist. Young adults frequently complain that, because the nursing staff does not follow their doctors' instructions on morphine dosages, they have suffered undue and unnecessary pain as a result.

'I believe that people with severe pain should receive appropriate, effective and adequate pain relief, including opiates (narcotics) if that is what is required; and that this assistance, which is generally given to terminal patients, should not be denied to those who may live many years with their pain and the illness that causes it,' writes one patient.

Epilogue

How We Can Help

Most of us are touched by pain sometime in our lives. We lose a parent or a grandparent, we nurse a sick child, someone in the family is diagnosed with a life-threatening illness, and we suffer the bereavement of friends and loved ones. Our relationships may fail, there will be the pain of divorce. Or the worst: we lose a child. We may learn that we have been diagnosed with a life-threatening illness ourselves.

As a teacher of children with physical and emotional disabilities, I witnessed and counselled families suffering greatly from abuse, misunderstanding, mis-diagnoses, lack of treatment, or living in fear and dread of the unknown. It is important to recognise that pain often comes with other physical symptoms. Emotional pain is also part and parcel of physiological pain — one should not be considered in isolation from the other. Emotional pain *is pain* and must be recognised and respected as such.

Words like cancer and tumour no longer come with the certainty of imminent death and are discussed much more openly than they used to be. As more books are written on the subject and as more doctors are willing to openly share their prognosis with their patients, some of your fear dissipates. But you need to know what you have to ask. You need strategies for coping with your worst nightmares. You are afraid of failure, of your own feelings.

Shifting the focus away from your own pain and worries, even when you are sick, is one of the ways in which you learn to deal with suffering. Self-absorption is not unusual when you are ill — it is so easy to think of nothing outside of your own problems. When your children are ill, hospitalised with leukaemia, suffering daily blood transfusions, undergoing the unimaginable procedure to have tumours removed and enduring constant painful if necessary treatments, you hurt in your whole body as you observe their sufferings and wish to take these upon yourself so that they may be pain-free. Impossible though this is, you can learn strategies — how to distract them, to comfort them and to ease their pain — to bring quality to their lives and to make each day matter.

Hospitals are much more aware of the healing presence of families and friends within the ward. Not only does it help the patient, but the nursing staff, always overworked, welcome the extra pair of hands: the person available to read a story to a child who is overwhelmed with pain or to sit with any patient who may lack a visitor himself that day.

The American surgeon Bernie Siegel learned much from his own patients who formed a group they called 'ECaP', or exceptional cancer patients. Siegel suggests that 'in the listening is the power': it is through listening that you can express your concerns, be it to a confidant, friend or therapist who only has to listen. At times there is no need even to speak. Sometimes just explaining how you feel by saying it out loud to others clarifies a lot of things. This is the reason why self-help groups become powerful: when you share your pain and your problems, you heal yourself. Families and friends often feel they cannot cure your problem, that they have nothing to offer and are useless. But by listening, hugging, holding hands, they are doing something to help.

Your friends and associates, often those you don't know very well, are able to help too. Why else would there be so much success with the 24-hour telephone help lines throughout the world, like those run by the Salvation Army, Lifeline and various religious missions. The staff is trained to listen, to refer and to offer comfort. These services seem to work because the callers feel safer confiding their hopelessness to anonymous strangers who they cannot see.

Late one evening while I was on night duty at SBSTV, the government-funded Australian television station, I received a telephone call from a Spanish woman. She sounded very weak and yet I could hear frantic despair in her voice. She said she had taken an overdose and knew she was going to die. But then, glancing at her television screen, she noticed we were broadcasting a Spanish program. Hearing her own language brought her comfort and it gave her the idea she might find someone at the television station with whom she could speak in her native tongue.

Quickly I beckoned to one of our Spanish team, who talked to the woman and found out her name and address so we could summon an ambulance. The Spanish subtitler talked calmly for fifteen minutes until she heard the ambulance officer entering the flat. We followed up the story through the ambulance service the next morning. The voice on the phone visited the grateful woman with a bunch of flowers and our best wishes for her to experience a happier life. This was a very enriching night for us all and led to discussions about how we could set up a service that would link us up with translators to cover the twenty-four hours. I believe that such a service still exists. This is one story with a reasonable outcome. If the person at the end of the phone (or by the bedside) is able to appear calm and confident, some of that control will in turn give comfort to the person in pain.

When you share your pain and problems with others, you all feel better. The mistake is to take the omnipotent view that you will be your own healer, the one responsible for some amazing shrinking of a tumour or for solving some other kind of crisis.

If you take the word 'patient' in its literal Latin meaning of 'submissive sufferer', you may make the error of seeing yourself as a victim. But you also have to take charge of your own healing and ask questions, even if it means being considered a 'difficult' patient. Rather, you are simply using your natural instinct for self-preservation and, if it challenges your treating physicians, that's an experience from which everyone may benefit.

When you are sick, you lose power. You are not yourself. Sometimes your illness knocks you down really badly and it is difficult to challenge authority. It is often easier to take the victim role, to be acquiescent. Be strong. If this book gives you even one idea along those lines, it will have served its purpose.

Humour has a role. Indeed, some practitioners have proved the value of taking on the role of clown doctors in children's wards, of watching and reading comedy. One of the sad symptoms of illness is often a loss-of-humour disorder and you may need to chivvy yourself and your friends.

One day I watched how a group of cerebral palsied children reacted when they observed the shadows of visiting medical students peering at them through the two-way mirror to their ward. 'Let's go all spazzy at them,' said Mark the ringleader, encouraging the others to make gestures he considered the students would associate with the cerebral palsied victim: flaying their arms up in the air in a bizarre manner and yelling incomprehensible words, then dropping their heads as if in death, on their chests in their wheelchairs. Only their laughter gave them away. As Mark said to me, 'If they want to gawk at us, then we give them something worth gawking at!' It's easy to forget, with all disabled people, that it is they who have every right to laugh at us.

It's great to smile more, to lighten up, just as it is right to ask for help. But how hesitant we are, fearing to let ourselves go, fearing 'being a nuisance'.

Four mothers I interviewed found great comfort from each other. Their children all had leukaemia, and endured blood transfusions five times a week, constant difficulty with the insertion of canulas, many tears and temper tantrums and much unhappiness. One morning the mothers were having a break and telling jokes. They were exploding with laughter at one particularly obscene tale when a pompous social worker walked in. 'How dare you all sit there laughing while your children are suffering so much,' she said. From that day forth, one of the mothers told me later, they restricted their dealings with the social worker to polite greetings. They felt she had no comprehension of their suffering. They had devised their own coping mechanisms and when they grieved, they preferred to do it at night, in private.

It is an attractive but totally unrealistic thought to imagine a world without pain. But learning to take a more positive attitude is important. I, myself, am only able to cope with pain some of the time, with the help of dedicated medical staff and with the kindness of my friends. A multi-disciplinary approach is the best road to take and this is often found all under one roof in a pain clinic. Coping is a team effort, and may have to be life-long.

Useful Web Addresses

Acupuncture

British Acupuncture Council:
www.acupuncture.org.uk
British Medical Acupuncture Society:
www.medical-acupuncture.co.uk
Acupuncture schools worldwide:
www.acufinder.com/search_schools.php

Alexander technique

www.alexandertechnique.com

Arachnoiditis

www.arachnoiditis.co.uk
Click on 'home' then 'links' for international addresses.
A good UK site: **www.patient.co.uk/showdoc/127**

Art therapy

British Association of Art Therapists: **www.baat.org**
International: **www.art-therapy.us/links**

Best-practice guidelines

**www.library.nhs.uk/guidelinesfinder/ViewResource.
aspx?resID=121392**
www.oqp.med.va.gov/cpg/cpg.htm

Chiropractic

For worldwide information visit **www.wfc.org**

Drug Regulatory Agency

en.wikipedia.org/wiki/Regulation_of_therapeutic_goods
You can then choose your country of interest.

Feldenkrais

www.feldenkrais.co.uk

Hospices and Respite Care

There are many websites that can be visited. A good place to start
is **www.hospicecare.com**

I have already told you about Helen House and Douglas House
www.helenanddouglas.org.uk

You may wish to consult **www.buddhanet.net/sitemap.htm**

For specific respite care information, if you are interested in what
the UK can offer, visit **www.nhsdirect.nhs.uk/articles/article.
aspx?articleId=537&sectionId=4**

Multiple Sclerosis

The main site is **www.mssociety.org.uk** for the UK and
www.msassociation.org for the USA.
An excellent international organisation is **www.msif.org**

Music Therapy

In the UK: **www.bsmt.org**
In the USA: **www.musictherapy.org**
Also recommended: **www.internationalsuzuki.org**

Osteopathy

Check out **www.osteopathy.org** or internationally **www.oialliance.org**

Pain Management

There are many sites devoted to the treatment of pain, some belonging to medical societies, others to private clinics. You can maybe go to **www.britishpainsociety.org/about_home.htm** or **www.pain.com**

Pets as Therapy

The excellent UK site is **www.petsastherapy.org**

Prolotherapy

For information on this alternative treatment:
www.drreevesonline.com/index.html or
www.prolotherapy.com

Psychiatrists

I recommend that you consult only practising psychiatrists who are members of their national society,:
www.rcpsych.ac.uk
www.psych.org

Psychologists

As with psychiatrists, I recommend you only consult members of your national society:
www.bps.org.uk or **www.apa.org**

RSI/OOS

Many excellent resources concerning RSI can be found in libraries and on the internet. A particularly useful author and website is Dr Robin McKenzie: **www.mckenziemdt.org**

You may also wish to consult **www.patient.co.uk/leaflets/ occupational_overuse_syndrome.htm**

Bernie Siegel

The US physician has written many valuable books on ways of coping with cancer **www.ecap-online.org**

Travelling

You will need to consult your own government website and if available also the website of the government of your destination country. **www.fco.gov.uk/en/travelling-and-living-overseas/ staying-safe/health**
http://seniors-site.com/travel/health.html
http://wwwn.cdc.gov/travel

Yoga

I recommend you seek a qualified yoga teacher.

www.yogauk.com/teachers/teachers.htm

www.yogasite.com/teacher_directory/teachers.php

References and Reading

You may have to ask your treating doctors to obtain papers published in medical journals for you, or you could find them in the printed journals at a medical library (at a university or hospital). .

Attitudes to opioids

Jane E Brody, 'Misunderstood prescription drugs and needless pain', *New York Times*, 22 January 2002. 'Far too little has been done to correct the misunderstandings of both patients and doctors that stand in the way of using opioids to control chronic pain.' Available at www.nytimes.com; you need to register to read the article, but it is free.

Jim Brown, 'Pain management with opiates', *Ivanhoe Broadcast News*, 30 January 1997; archived at http://www.masmith.inspired. net.au/pain/opiates.htm: 'Every year, thousands of people suffer needlessly and many commit suicide because they cannot get treatment for pain.'

Robert Carlson, 'Risk of addiction to pain relief is small, expert says', report of address at the American Academy of Emergency Medicine annual meeting, February 2000, on the *Doctor's Guide* website (www.docguide.com): 'Most pain experts say the public's concern about inadvertently becoming addicted to narcotics while being treated for pain is unfounded. Unfortunately, some physicians share that concern, and some patients are not getting the pain relief they need.'

Fibroworld's *The Opioid Controversy* (http://members.aol.com/ imagine524/opioid.htm) includes the paper David E Joranson *et. al*, 'Tolerance, physical dependence, and psychological dependence (addiction)' and good links.

Judy Hall, letter to US Congress. According to www.masmith. inspired.net.au: 'Judy wrote this letter about the 'Pain Patient Crisis' and sent it to the women of the Congress and Senate in August 2001, … it seems those in Washington put it aside or didn't read it. Not long after mailing her letter, in November 2001, Judy found that she couldn't live with her pain any longer … and took her own life.' The full text of Judy Hall's letter to Congress is at http://www.cpmission.com/main/painpolitics/polarticles/judyh. html.

C. Stratton Hill Jr, 'When will adequate pain treatment be the norm?', *Journal of the American Medical Association*, editorial, 20 December 1995, vol 274 no 23 p 1881; available at http:// members.aol.com/imagine524/painabstr.htm: 'Patients should demand appropriate pain relief in light of evidence showing that few hospital patients become addicted to painkillers.'

Alexis Jetter, 'The end of pain: now there's a pill that can safely ease every agony from cancer to a bad back — so why are doctors and patients afraid of it?'; archived at http://www.masmith. inspired.net.au/. This article discusses the use of morphine and methadone for chronic pain, and especially the work of neurosurgeon James Campbell, who runs the pain clinic at Johns Hopkins Hospital. Methadone is a very special case of a useful medication with an unholy stigma: a story worth telling in itself.

'Making gains on chronic pain', *Medical Journal of Australia*, press release dated 5 January 2003 about the poor treatment of pain among nursing home residents in rural New South Wales. A survey has shown that older people are suffering pain unnecessarily and too many of them are not being offered pain relief medications at all. Available at http://www.ama.com.au/ web.nsf/ doc/WEEN-5HH4J2.

Ronald Melzack, 'The tragedy of needless pain', *Scientific American*, February 1990; available at www.masmith.inspired.net.au/pain/ tragedy.htm: 'Contrary to popular belief … morphine taken solely to control pain is not addictive. Yet patients worldwide continue to be undertreated and to suffer unnecessary agony.'.

'Morphine as Medicine', transcript of CNN/Time Impact story (broadcast 6 April 1997), archived at http://www.masmith. inspired.net.au/pain/impact.htm.

D. Moulin, 'Opioid analgesics in the management of neuropathic pain', *Pain Research & Management*, Spring 2000, vol 5, no 1, pp 89–91; abstract available at http://www.pulsus.com/Pain/05_01/

moul_ed.htm: 'Psychological dependence or addiction ... is not usually an issue in pain management with opioid analgesics. The extant literature strongly suggests the trial of an opioid analgesic in the management of neuropathic pain if adjuvant analgesics fail to provide adequate pain control. Failure of one opioid warrants a trial of another opioid because their effectiveness can vary among patients; the results are based on physiochemical properties of the drug and idiosyncratic reactions of the patient. Neuropathic pain can be a difficult problem to manage, and sometimes the use of an opioid analgesic can make the difference between bearable and unbearable pain so that patients can get on with their lives.'

'Politics of Heroin', transcript of the ABC's *Four Corners* program (broadcast 1 April 2002). Describes how Prime Minister John Howard put the Salvation Army in charge of the war against drugs and opposed an Australian prescription heroin trial.

Sierra Sacramento Valley Medical Society, 'The painful dilemma: the use of narcotics for the treatment of chronic pain', 1990; available at http://www.ssvms.org/resource/pain.asp: 'Evidence is steadily accumulating that persons with intractable pain do not respond to narcotics in the same way as do street addicts. Their motivations are different, and so are their psychological reactions and tolerances to the drugs. The pain patient can be treated with narcotics with little risk of developing the self-destructive behavior characteristic of addiction.'

Jacob Sullum, 'No relief in sight', in *Reason* magazine (January

1997), available at http://www.reason.com/news/show/30113. html: 'Torture, despair, agony, and death are the symptoms of "opiophobia", a well-documented medical syndrome fed by fear, superstition, and the war on drugs. Doctors suffer the syndrome. Patients suffer the consequences.'

Anne-Marie Vidal, 'The Politics of Pain: The controversy surrounding chronic pain and opioids', 2002; available at http:// www.ourfm-cfidsworld.org/html/the_politics_of_pain.html. This article is a review of recent events: 'Anyone who lives with chronic pain is acutely aware of many physicians' difficulty in coming to terms with prescribing adequate pain medication. For us, this is more than a research or academic issue. We know first hand that pain is debilitating and can erode our standard of living and ability to earn an income. ... We live in an era where our right to adequate pain relief is recognized but continuously challenged.'

'A World of Pain': a transcript of ABC (Australia) Radio National *Background Briefing* documentary about chronic pain treatment (broadcast 5 December 2004). Helen Thomas interviewed pain patients, doctors and researchers about their attitudes to opioid drugs: '... doctors worry about prescribing them, patients fret about taking them, and we all buy into the stigma that surrounds them. The end result is a widespread lack of pain relief, an under-management of pain that some describe as a national crisis.' See www.abc.net.au.

Attitudes to pain

Marcia E. Bedard, 'Bankruptcies of the heart: secondary losses from disabling chronic pain' dispels the myth of 'secondary gain': 'The basic idea behind this theory is that chronic pain is psychological and persists only because the person suffering from it enjoys one or more "rewards" that accrue from their pain. These so-called "rewards" may be emotional, such as sympathy — or monetary, such as disability payments.' Summary available on www.cssa-inc.org/Articles/Bankruptcies.htm. See also Marcia Bedard's 'Chronic pain fact sheet'; also on the website of the Chronic Syndrome Support Association (www.cssa-inc.org).

Frank Fisher, 'Chronic pain and opioids: debunking the myths', from *Our Chronic Pain Mission* website; available at http://www. cpmission.com/main/debunk.html.

Marilyn Oakes, 'Countering chronic pain myths', available at www.arachnoiditis.info: 'When representing chronic pain patients, attorneys must counter the chronic pain myths.' A certified pain practitioner gives advice to lawyers on how to rebuff the arguments put by 'the other side' in insurance and disability cases.

Robert W. Teasell, 'The denial of chronic pain', *Pain Research & Management*, Summer 1997, vol 2, no 2, editorial; at http://www. pulsus.com/pain/02_02/teas_ed.htm: 'There is a current disconcerting trend towards dealing with chronic pain and its subsequent disability by denying its reality. The reason for this has primarily been cost containment and cost reduction.' This article argues against the 'rehabilitation model described in Moira A Smith, 'Know your enemy: personal observations on the rehabilitation model of chronic pain' (available at http://www.masmith.inspired. net.au/pain/enemy.htm), which is beloved of insurers.

Ellen Thompson, 'Back pain: bankrupt expertise and new directions', *Pain Research & Management*, Winter 1997, vol 2, no 4, editorial; available at http://www.pulsus.com/Pain/02_04/thom_ ed.htm: 'Bankrupt experts operate with the faulty assumption that pain not seen on x-rays or scans, nor cured by surgery, was "nonorganic", equalling "psychosomatic" or "psychogenic" (which in many jurisdictions is noncompensable).'

Cannabis

'Cannabis from the chemist', available at http://www.abc.net. au/4corners/stories/s511147.htm. This is a link from the website of the Australian ABC, which broadcast a *Four Corners* report on the topic (on 25 March 2002), including the use of cannabis for chronic pain. Further research is being carried out in hospitals to make cannabis available in pill form so that those who dislike the notion of smoking may obtain the benefits of pain relief.

Statements and position papers

American Academy of Pain Medicine and the American Pain Society, 'The use of opioids for the treatment of chronic pain,' consensus statement, 1996; available at http://www.ampainsoc. org/advocacy/opioids.htm: 'The undertreatment of pain in today's society is not justified.'

American Society of Addiction Medicine, 'Rights and responsibilities of healthcare professionals in the use of opioids for the treatment of pain', public policy statement, April 1997; available at http://www.ampainsoc.org/advocacy/rights.htm: 'Healthcare professional (HCP) concerns regarding the potential for harm to patients, as well as possible legal, regulatory, licensing or other third party sanctions related to the prescription of opioids, contribute significantly to the mistreatment of pain.'

Canadian Pain Society Taskforce, 'Use of opioid analgesics for the treatment of chronic noncancer pain', consensus statement and guidelines, *Pain Research & Management*, 1998, vol 3, no 4; available at http://www.pulsus.com/Pain/03_04/opio_ed.htm: 'Pain of all types is undertreated in our society ... Physicians' fears of using opioid therapy, and the fears of other health professionals, contribute to this problem.'

'Europe against Pain', news of an initiative to educate European Union decision makers and health professionals about chronic pain issues. See www.europeanpainnetwork.com.

Paul Graziotti and Roger Goucke, 'The use of oral opioids in patients with chronic non-malignant pain', Australian Pain Society position paper; available at www.apsoc.org.au/pdfs/opiods/pdf. '[M]any doctors may decide not to prescribe opioids for patients with chronic non-malignant pain ... Worldwide though there is a growing body of opinion that a small sub-group of patients with chronic non-malignant pain may improve their level of function whilst achieving improved analgesia in the absence of rapidly escalating doses and/or behaviour.'

Pain and Symptom Management Task Force, *Report to the Seventieth Oregon Legislative Assembly and Governor John Kitzhaber*, January 1999, available at www.myalgia.com. Recommendations include the adoption of a resolution of rights for persons with pain, and better education for health-care providers.

On Dr William Hurwitz and legal issues

Hurwitz, an American pain management doctor, was convicted of 'drug trafficking' in OxyContin because some of his patients misused medication he prescribed. The conviction was later overturned. At the time of writing, Dr Hurwitz was being retried. The subject has been widely explored on websites and in print.

William Hurwitz, 'Pain Control in The Police State of Medicine, Part II', *Journal of American Physicians and Surgeons,* Spring 2003; also available at http://www.jpands.org/vol8no1/hurwitz.pdf. Hurwitz explains why he has decided to stop practising medicine in the USA.

William Hurwitz, 'The Police State of Medicine', address to the Drug Policy Foundation in New Orleans, 18 October 1997: 'I was charged with having prescribed excessive doses of opioid analgesics in the treatment of 30 patients who, it was acknowledged by the Board of Medicine, had conditions causing intractable pain.

William Hurwitz, The Police State of Medicine: Reflections on a Case of Regulatory Abuse, *Medical Sentinel,* 1998, vol 3, no 4, pp 131–33; this is also available at www.aapsonline.org/painman/hurwitz.htm.

Damien Cave, 'No Relief', *Salon* online magazine (published 11 April 2002): 'Increasing numbers of the estimated 30 to 50 million people in the country who suffer from some form of chronic pain say the OxyContin crackdown means they can no longer get adequate or sustained relief.'

Terri Roberts, 'OxyContin problem not that complicated'. Roberts, of the About Headaches & Migranes website (www.headaches.about.com), discusses recent developments and introduces an article from *MAGNUM*, the National Migraine Association's magazine (published March 2002). 'The OxyContin issue has produced an aggressive public health policy that would limit access to those in pain from receiving appropriate pain management. Furthermore, discussions at recent hearings could lead to very tight control over what pain medications doctors may prescribe in general. Doctors may choose not to treat those in debilitating pain for fear of being profiled and/or targeted by law enforcement or other monitoring state or federal agencies.'

Jacob Sullum, 'Healers and Dealers' in *Reason* magazine (19 November 2004), available at www.reason.com/news/35967.html. Discusses why Hurwitz faces a life sentence: 'Prosecuting doctors for their patients' misuse of narcotics hurts people in pain'.

The webpage http://www.aapsonline.org/painman/policestate. htm contains links to news and information about Dr Hurwitz's trial.

For more internet links, see 'Pain policy & law, the use of opioids in the treatment of chronic non-malignant pain' and other pages on Lois Randall's *Medical Information Network* site at http://www2. rpa.net/~lrandall/index.html.

Further reading

Eric J. Cassell, *The Nature of Suffering and the Goals of Medicine*, Oxford University Press, New York, 1994.

Norman Cousins, *The Celebration of Life: A Dialogue on Hope, Spirit and the Immortality of the Soul*, Bantam, New York, 1974.

Hilde Hemmes, *Herbs and Health with Hilde Hemmes*, Australian School of Herbal Medicine, Ridgehaven SA, 2003.

Deborah Hutton, *What Can I Do to Help?*, Short Books, London, 2005.

Elisabeth Kübler-Ross, *On Death and Dying*, Simon & Shuster, New York, 1969.

Leora Kuttner, *A Child in Pain: How to Help, What to Do*, Hartley & Marks, Point Roberts WA, 1996.

C.S. Lewis, *The Problem of Pain*, Geoffrey Bles/The Centenary Press, London, 1940.

William Livingston, *Pain and Suffering*, IASP Press, Seattle, 1998.

R.D. Mann (ed), *The History of the Management of Pain: From Early Principles to Present Practice*, Parthenon, Carnforth, 1988.

Harold Mersky, *et. al* (eds), *The Paths of Pain 1975–2005*, IASP Press, Seattle, 2005.

David B. Morris, *The Culture of Pain*, University of California Press, Berkeley, 1913.

Michael Nicholas *et. al*, *Manage Your Pain*, ABC Books, Sydney, 2000.

Bernie S. Siegel, *How to Live Between Office Visits*, HarperCollins, New York, 2001

Bernie S. Siegel, *Love, Medicine and Miracles*, HarperCollins, New York, 2001

Acknowledgements

I have been greatly assisted in the writing of this book by Dr Richard Hallinan, FAChAM (RACP), who has a special interest in chronic pain and addiction treatment, as well as having worked for years as a professional violinist. I extend my tremendous gratitude to him for his generosity. As well as assisting me with medical aspects, he has had a significant editorial contribution.

This book would not have been possible without the help of many organisations and individuals who have given unstintingly of their time, skill and dedication. In particular I wish to thank John Thompson, Lady Natasha Spender, David Champion, Tiina Jaaniste, Verena Clemencic-Jones, Erica Booker, Shirlie Andrews, Sally Jardine, Annette Leggo, Maureen Stephenson and the Alison Hunter Memorial Foundation for use of their material and web pages, Bernie Siegel for his inspiring words, Aaron McMillan for his courage and example, Robert Barker, Dame Joan Sutherland, Lizzie Pickering, Renée McCullough, Sister Frances, Helen House Oxford, Irina Dunn, Lesley McFadjean, Chris and Miffy Vaughan, Denise Park, Jan Cummings and the NSW Writers' Centre, and Mary Trewby for her sensitive and helpful editing. Many other people have influenced my life and inspired me to carry on writing a very demanding text. Over five years, I interviewed a hundred people and I thank those who wish to remain anonymous and who gave me full medical family histories (their names and conditions have been changed to protect their privacy), Marilyn Uebel, Vivienne Tedeschi, and the many friends who have plied me with meals and hot drinks to keep the show on the road. Thank you all.

I would like to emphasise that any errors that may have crept into the manuscript are entirely my own responsibility and not those of the many people who have kindly helped me along the road to publication.

Index